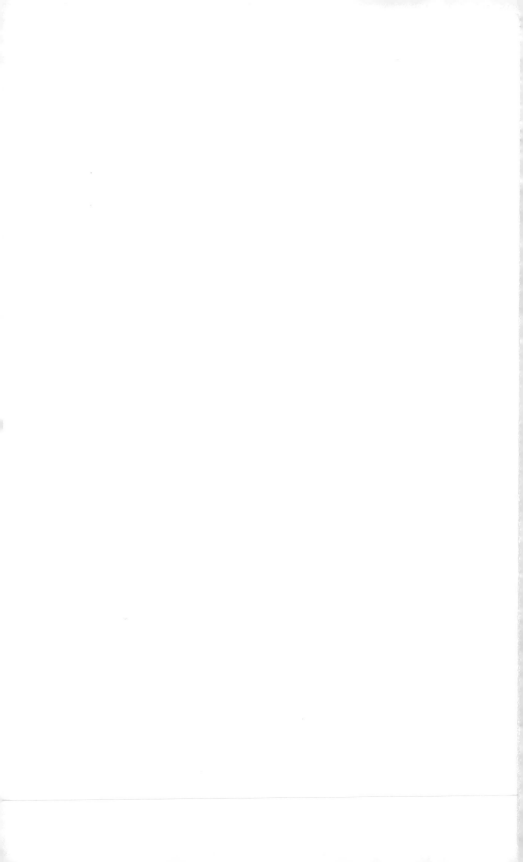

Detoxify

Detoxify

THE EVERYDAY TOXINS HARMING
YOUR IMMUNE SYSTEM AND
HOW TO DEFEND AGAINST THEM

ALY COHEN, MD

SIMON ELEMENT
NEW YORK   AMSTERDAM/ANTWERP   LONDON
TORONTO   SYDNEY/MELBOURNE   NEW DELHI

SIMON
ELEMENT

An Imprint of Simon & Schuster, LLC
1230 Avenue of the Americas
New York, NY 10020

Copyright © 2025 by Aly Cohen, MD

This publication contains the opinions and ideas of its author. It is intended to provide helpful and informative material on the subjects addressed in the publication. It is sold with the understanding that the author and publisher are not engaged in rendering medical, health, or any other kind of personal professional services in the book. The reader should consult his or her medical, health, or other competent professional before adopting any of the suggestions in this book or drawing inferences from it.

The author and publisher specifically disclaim all responsibility for any liability, loss, or risk, personal or otherwise, that is incurred as a consequence, directly or indirectly, of the use and application of any of the contents of this book.

Mention of websites, apps, or companies in this book does not imply endorsement by the author or publisher, nor does it imply that such companies or organizations have endorsed the author or publisher. Internet addresses given in the book were accurate at the time it went to press. The author and publisher are not responsible for changes to third-party websites.

All rights reserved, including the right to reproduce this book or portions thereof in any form whatsoever. For information, address Simon Element Subsidiary Rights Department, 1230 Avenue of the Americas, New York, NY 10020.

First Simon Element hardcover edition May 2025

SIMON ELEMENT is a trademark of Simon & Schuster, LLC

For information about special discounts for bulk purchases, please contact Simon & Schuster Special Sales at 1-866-506-1949 or business@simonandschuster.com.

The Simon & Schuster Speakers Bureau can bring authors to your live event. For more information or to book an event, contact the Simon & Schuster Speakers Bureau at 1-866-248-3049 or visit our website at www.simonspeakers.com.

Interior design by Matt Ryan

Manufactured in the United States of America

10 9 8 7 6 5 4 3 2 1

Library of Congress Cataloging-in-Publication Data has been applied for.

ISBN 978-1-6680-3353-1
ISBN 978-1-6680-3355-5 (ebook)

For my supportive parents, my amazing husband, my two beautiful sons,

and the community of environmental health warriors

who are fighting every day to make this world cleaner and safer for all of us.

The secret of change is to focus
all your energy not on fighting the old
but on building the new.

—Socrates

CONTENTS

Preface: User Guide to This Book and the 21-Day Plan — ix

Introduction — 1

SECTION I: ASSESS

Chapter 1: The Smoking Gun: Environmental Chemicals — 15

Chapter 2: Your Body on Chemicals — 33

Chapter 3: How and Why Dangerous Environmental Chemicals Exist — 69

SECTION II: AVOID

Chapter 4: What's Really in Your Water — 81

Chapter 5: What's Really in Your Food — 119

Chapter 6: What's Really in Your Personal-Care Products — 153

Chapter 7: What's Really Inside Your Home — 179

SECTION III: ADD

Chapter 8: Using Food to Detoxify — 205

Chapter 9: The Three Ss to Detoxify — 237

The *Detoxify* Plan: Twenty-One Days to Restore and Improve Your Health — 261

Appendix 1: 100 Top Detoxifying Foods to Add to Your Shopping Cart — 287

Appendix 2: Medical and Other Laboratory Testing — 293

Appendix 3: DIY Household Cleaners — 301

Appendix 4: Detox Recipes — 307

Appendix 5: Online Resources — 329

Acknowledgments — 333

Notes — 337

PREFACE

User Guide to This Book and the 21-Day Plan

BOTH THE CONTENT of both this book and the 21-Day Plan that begins on page 261 are structured in a strategic and sequential order of what I call the "four As"—*Assess, Avoid, Add, Allow*. What does this mean? When it comes to environmental chemicals, you want to *assess* before you *avoid*, *avoid* before you *add*, and *add* before you *allow*. While taking any action to better understand and mitigate your toxic load is important to your overall health, reading this book and following the 21-Day Plan in that order will help you make effective, strategic, and seamless changes to supercharge your body and overhaul your physical and mental health. Here's why.

Assess

You can't change what you don't know needs to be changed. Knowledge is key to combating environmental chemicals, which is why the first step in our journey—and the first three chapters of this book—are dedicated to assessing what you need to know about harmful environmental toxins, including what they are; why so many are allowed to exist in our food, water, homes, and personal-care products; and what they do to our bodies and health. Similarly, the first week of the 21-Day Plan is structured to help you assess your personal chemical exposures and identify any related symptoms so you can begin to address the problem at its source.

Avoid

Once you've assessed and identified the problem, you can start to avoid it—strategically, effectively, and successfully. That's why chapters 4 through 7 are devoted to teaching you what to do to avoid common chemicals in your food, water, home, and personal-care products. Once you know the science of "why," doing the "what" will make sense. Likewise, the second week of the 21-Day Plan shows you how to leverage what you assessed during week 1 so that you can take the most effective steps to reduce your specific points of exposure and any related symptoms.

Add

Only after you start to target and reduce your environmental exposure can you begin to take the extra measures that can ramp up your body's ability to detoxify. Otherwise, trying to boost your body's detoxifying powers can be counterproductive if you're still overloading it with chemicals from food, water, indoor air, and personal-care products. For this reason, chapters 8 and 9, which detail how to amplify the body's detoxifying abilities through science-backed steps, offer help after you've learned how to assess and avoid environmental chemicals, thus making any detoxifying steps you adopt more fruitful and effective. Similarly, the third week of the 21-Day Plan shows you how to adopt detoxifying strategies after you've assessed and avoided what you need to detoxify from.

Allow

The final step of your journey is allowing a new mindset or adopting a different perspective that helps you make what you've assessed, avoided, and added a permanent part of your life. This new mindset also teaches you how to allow for flexibility when encountering real-life situations, like those times when you can't avoid certain exposures while you're on vacation or at special events like parties or holidays—or if you want to continue to color your hair (like I do) or use a certain product you know contains chemicals in small or infrequent amounts, while limiting your exposure in other areas. So, at the end of the 21-Day Plan, you'll find the tips and tricks that will help you incorporate everything you've learned into your everyday life.

WHILE THERE'S RHYME and reason behind the structure of this book and the 21-Day Plan, you should feel free to explore areas that interest you the most and read them as often as you want. Consider this book and 21-Day Plan a resource for life, not one-and-done material. You can return to it repeatedly for more information, action steps, and solace. From personal experience, I know that once you begin to dig into the science of environmental chemicals and learn how to fight against them, it can be difficult to stop. That's because the journey you're about to embark upon removes any fears, frustrations, or feelings of being overwhelmed and replaces them with action, empowerment, and, perhaps most important, results you can see and feel. So, get ready: you're about to change your life.

Introduction

SOMETIMES, OUR GREATEST gains come as a result of our biggest losses. If it weren't for the death of my beloved four-year-old golden retriever Truxtun in 2008, I might not have written this book. I also might not have gone on the extensive journey I did, both professionally and personally, to become one of the few medical doctors in the world who understands the impact environmental toxins can have on human health, along with what we can do, both practically and sustainably, to mitigate or even reverse those impacts and prevent or treat various symptoms and diseases.

Also, as a dog lover, I believe every good story starts with a good pup.

Shortly after we were married, my husband and I adopted Truxtun from a breeder in Pennsylvania, and we moved into an old farmhouse perched on the edge of acres of farmland outside the university town of Princeton, New Jersey. The house was rustic and lovely, with a big back porch and lots of lawn, which seemed perfect for a puppy—or so we thought. True to point, Truxtun at first appeared happy and lively in our new home, living up to his namesake: eighteenth-century naval officer Thomas Truxtun, one of the first captains to command a ship in the US Navy. Like Truxtun the officer, Truxtun the dog loved the water, in addition to chewing on everything he could find, from shoes and furniture to sticks and the siding of our home. But his biggest chew obsession was a red plastic dog toy, which he constantly kept in his mouth, not even releasing it from his slobbery grasp when he slept at night.

Four years into his puppyhood, something changed, though. Truxtun started to pant heavily, which at first we assumed was normal dog stuff. We continued to monitor him, but with a two-and-a-half-year-old toddler and a six-month-old infant at home, plus our full-time jobs, my husband and I didn't have a ton of time to focus on anything other than diaper changes, feeding duties, and maximizing our sleep. After all, I had to be as sharp as possible when I saw patients.

When Truxton refused to eat, however, I knew something was wrong. What dog doesn't scarf down everything in sight? I took him to the vet, who, after a quick physical exam, concluded there was nothing wrong with him and sent us home, frustrated and vexed. (Sound familiar? The same thing happens all the time with human patients, who get told by doctors that there's nothing wrong, even when the patient knows or suspects otherwise. In this book, I'll help you better navigate that problem, if you've ever experienced it.)

The day after we took Truxtun to the vet, he flopped down in the middle of the kitchen, refusing to get up even after my husband and I both tripped over him repeatedly and our two young sons started pulling on his fur. The following morning, I took him back to the same clinic and asked to see a different vet, who immediately noticed the inside of his ears were yellow—an indication of a possible liver problem. The vet then ordered blood work, a chest X-ray, and an ultrasound of his abdomen. From these tests, we discovered that Truxtun's liver had shrunk to the size of a tennis ball—so small it could no longer function, let alone function optimally.

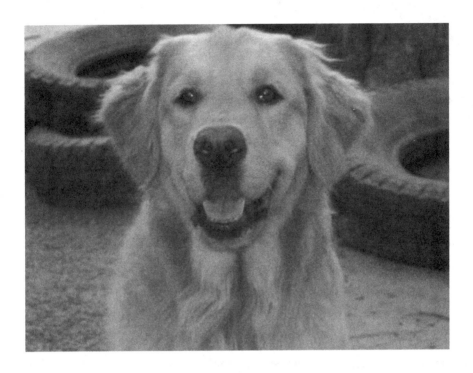

What could cause Truxtun's liver to shrivel to the point of collapse? The most likely reason, the vet said, was that Truxton had an autoimmune liver disease. Autoimmune diseases—a category that includes common conditions like rheumatoid arthritis, inflammatory bowel disease, and Hashimoto's thyroiditis—occur when the body's immune system begins to attack healthy cells, not just the unhealthy ones and foreign "invaders" like bad bacteria and viruses.

I was shocked. Here I was, a board-certified rheumatologist—a doctor who specializes in diagnosing and treating inflammatory conditions like autoimmune disease—and it didn't even occur to me that my own dog could have what I saw so often in patients, many who were just like Truxton: suffering from an autoimmune illness at a relatively young age.

At the same time, autoimmune liver disease is very rare in dogs—and even more so in golden retrievers. This caused me a lot of concern: if the illness is so rare in dogs, why did my young dog develop the disease? As a doctor, I've long believed in the power of detective work to get to the bottom of what's really wrong with my human patients, and I knew I needed to apply that same approach with my dog.

MY FIRST INSTINCT was to call the breeder, whom my husband and I had researched extensively to ensure there was a history of rearing dogs responsibly and ethically. I wasn't surprised, then, when the breeder told me neither Truxtun's mom, sire, nor any pup from that litter had health issues, let alone liver problems. The breeder had also never seen or heard of an autoimmune liver disease in a golden retriever, which, along with the vet's opinion, seemed to rule out family history or a congenital problem.

I next considered what Truxtun was eating. Maybe his food was contaminated—toxins in dog food had just started to make headlines that year—so we changed brands, then began making his food from scratch, even though neither of us really had time. Germane to this book, however, is something I truly believe: *When you care enough about your health or someone else's, you can find time, because good health, especially when you realize it may be in jeopardy, is the most valuable thing we can do, buy, or experience.*

I then thought about what Truxtun was drinking. We had always filled his water bowl from the tap, and while I didn't know much about environmental toxins at the time, I was concerned how the chemicals routinely sprayed on the farmlands around our home might affect our groundwater and, by proxy, our drinking water. For this reason, I had started buying bottled water for my family, believing at the time it was healthier than tap water (spoiler alert: it's not). I started pouring bottled water into Truxtun's bowl.

The more factors I considered in Truxtun's disease development, the more I began to research the role environmental toxins might have played in aggravating, if not causing, his condition. I thought, for example, about the red chew toy he loved so much and whether all the plastic he was ingesting by chewing it all day could have helped to induce an autoimmune disease. Then, I considered the tick and flea medicine I regularly rubbed into Truxtun's fur: if the medicine could kill insects on contact, what might it do to animal cells after being absorbed by the skin? The same went for his heartworm medication: could that interfere with his immune system function or damage his liver cells while also killing parasites? Finally, I thought about our back porch and lawn, where Truxtun loved to lie and play. These were covered in pesticide residue anytime the local farmers sprayed the fields near our home. While I didn't realize it at the time, what I was doing was collecting an environmental-exposure history for my dog, something I would eventually begin doing with all my patients.

Every time I learned how chemicals might affect an animal's immune system or trigger some disease, I modified Truxtun's routine. At the same time, I knew whatever changes we made wouldn't be enough: by the time we discovered our dog was sick, his autoimmune condition was so advanced it was irreversible. The only thing we could do was make Truxton as comfortable as possible, giving him steroids and other medications to help "quiet" his immune system. Every night, we also drained large amounts of thick amber fluid from Truxtun's abdomen using long needles, intravenous tubing, and plastic IV bags.

Six months after Truxtun was diagnosed, we realized his pain and discomfort greatly outweighed the options we had to manage them. Finally, we made the difficult decision to relieve his suffering, knowing it would be better for our dog than living in constant pain and agony. In the vet's office, Truxtun gave us each a big lick across our faces before our "first child" succumbed to an illness no one could understand how he had developed in the first place.

After Truxtun died, I was heartbroken—so much so that I knew I had to channel my grief somehow. And it was easy to find a place for my agitation: piqued by all the research I'd read and angry that I hadn't learned anything about environmental toxins in med school, I continued to search for answers as to why my dog got sick and whether common chemicals may have played a role. At the time, the research on the impact of environmental toxins on human and animal health was still relatively nascent, but despite this, I found dozens of studies linking common chemicals in food, water, personal-care products, furniture, and other everyday items with disruptions of the endocrine system—the body's network of organs, glands, and tissues that regulates and controls the hormones responsible for growth, reproduction, metabolism, and other critical functions. Endocrine disruption, in turn, has been strongly associated with causing a host of health problems, including weight gain, infertility, depression, thyroid problems, neurological disease, learning problems in children, genitalia changes in newborns, heart and breathing troubles, and hormone-sensitive cancers, in addition to other health issues.

The more I learned about environmental toxins, the more I began to realize that endocrine-disrupting chemicals (EDCs), as they're known, were just the tip of the iceberg. Many EDCs don't just interfere with hormone function and expression; they also disrupt the normal function of the body's immune system—reducing our immunity, stoking chronic inflammation, and triggering abnormal immune responses like those that can cause autoimmune conditions. The research connecting environmental toxins to lowered immunity, inflammatory changes, and poor immune function was so overwhelming, in fact, that I eventually coined the term *immune-disrupting chemicals* (IDCs) to describe the devastating effect toxins can have on the body's immune system.

Armed with this new knowledge, I began to make changes in what my family and I ate, drank, and slathered, sprayed, or otherwise put in or on our bodies, all to help lower our toxin exposure. Almost immediately, these changes reversed the migraine headaches I had suffered from for years. I watched in real time as other aspects of my family's health began to improve, too (the specifics of which I'll share later in this book). Inspired, I continued to make other changes, like swapping our conventional cleaning supplies and furniture for cleaner versions and taking other targeted steps to make my home as "clean" as possible without breaking the bank.

A few years after Truxtun died, I took another critical step in my journey. Already a double board-certified internist and rheumatologist, I decided to become a board-certified doctor of integrative medicine. *Integrative medicine* is an approach to healing that considers all aspects of a patient's health and lifestyle, including environmental exposure, to help prevent illness before it occurs and to treat disease at its root cause. As the name suggests, integrative medicine blends the best of Western medicine, like using life-saving procedures and prescription medications (when necessary) with the ancient practices and evidence-based lifestyle changes of Eastern medicine. Influenced by my training with Dr. Andrew Weil at the Arizona Center for Integrative Medicine, I began to dig deeper into the health problems associated with everyday chemicals and the steps we can take to reduce toxin-related illnesses and improve our body's ability to detoxify.

EVENTUALLY, I APPLIED my training and experience to my patients—many of whom, like Truxtun, were experiencing symptoms or diseases at a young age for which they had no family history. In addition to medical histories, I started collecting environmental-exposure histories for all my patients (which no other doctor I knew at the time was doing). I also began ordering lab work that would assess their blood and urine for nutrient levels and common toxins—tests underutilized by conventional doctors, even though these labs are covered by most health insurance policies. This is why I say I do "detective work" when I see patients: I do everything I can and collect all possible data points to get to the bottom of what might be causing their symptoms.

For all my patients, I also prescribe diet, lifestyle, and product changes that often relieve, treat, or even reverse their symptoms—in addition to ordering blood work and any necessary diagnostic tests. As an integrative doctor, I know this is another way I'm unique among conventional physicians trained only in Western medicine: I try to *prevent* disease before it occurs, rather than treat the symptoms and illnesses after patients are already sick and the metaphorical horse has left the stable. And I prevent disease using evidence-based medicine that shows how boosting our overall nutrition and reducing our environmental exposure can help reduce and reverse symptoms— areas that conventional medicine chooses to ignore.

I'm not only frustrated with the conventional medical system: I'm also outraged at manufacturers and the government, which allow tens of thousands of chemicals to exist in our food, water, personal-care products, and other everyday items, even though most of these chemicals have *never* even been tested for human safety. Like many Americans, I used to assume that if I could buy something in a grocery store, pharmacy, or big-box retailer, it had undergone regulatory checks and was proven to be safe. Now I know better: very few chemicals are regulated by the government, even those shown to be dangerous to human health.[1] What's more, when products are found to harm consumers, their removal from store shelves is entirely up to the manufacturer, which may or may not comply. Making matters worse, many common chemicals interfere with our health in only small doses, overturning the age-old premise that "the dose makes the poison." And when it comes to new-age chemicals, very few age-old adages apply, and anything goes in today's Wild West of toxic compounds; these chemicals are ubiquitous in many products, including those considered "healthy" or even labeled "all-natural" or "organic."

For these reasons, I wrote the book *Non-Toxic: Guide to Living Healthy in a Chemical World* with renowned chemical expert Frederick S. vom Saal.² *Non-Toxic* focused squarely on the hormone health effects of everyday chemicals, known as *endocrine disruptors*, and what readers could do to avoid these effects. Now, I'm ready to do more with this book, introducing readers to how IDCs and EDCs greatly influence and can even change our health.

Here are some truths about IDCs that you'll learn in this book:

- Chemicals that affect the immune system are ubiquitous.
- Chemicals can be absorbed by our skin, lungs, gastrointestinal tract, and vaginal and anal mucosa, and even cross the placenta to affect an unborn child.
- Low-level exposure to IDCs over time and/or during vulnerable periods of human development (as in childhood) can significantly raise the risk for illness.
- Exposures to IDCs have the potential to change our genetic expression—changes that may affect the health of not only our children but also future generations.
- Disorders of the immune system linked to IDCs have become epidemic.
- There is nearly *no* regulation of IDCs in products sold or manufactured in the United States.
- There are so many ways to lower your exposure to IDCs, thereby reducing the risk of illness; these methods are simple, accessible, and inexpensive.

The good news is that simple changes, like those you'll learn about in this book, can go a long way toward reducing your chemical exposure and alleviating any symptoms and diseases associated with environmental toxins. Every day as a doctor, I see significant improvements in my patients' health when they make the same changes as you'll find in this book. I've also taught thousands of students in high schools, colleges, medical schools, and even physician-training programs about the environmental toxins. And from these young people and my patients, I've seen firsthand how exciting it can be when people learn they can make simple changes in real time that actually improve their health.

I'm living proof that it's never too late to make a difference. When Truxtun got sick, I was drinking diet soda, eating processed foods, using toxic cleaning supplies, and spritzing, smearing, and rubbing chemical-laden personal-care products all over my body. Today, I've cleaned up my diet, changed my personal-care routine, and altered my lifestyle without spending a ton of money or sacrificing my favorite foods or products, or even abstaining from doing the things I enjoy most. I still color my hair with a chemical dye, and I occasionally use or consume items that contain known toxins. The goal of this book isn't to be perfect: *it's to be as healthy as possible without losing your mind, your money, or your sense of well-being.*

IN THE FOLLOWING pages, you'll learn the surprising ways in which environmental toxins influence the body and what symptoms and illnesses are closely associated with everyday exposures. You'll also read patient stories that may sound similar to yours—people who have struggled for months, years, or even decades with the same symptoms, without getting the answers they deserve. And you'll hear how they were able to treat their condition by reducing their environmental exposure, while improving their bodies' ability to detoxify.

Additionally, you'll also discover what's in your water, food, personal-care products, and other household goods. Equally important, you'll find out what you can do, simply and inexpensively, to live a more toxin-free life. You'll get to decide which sacrifices are worth the effort, and which ones may not make sense for your lifestyle or budget. You'll also discover the specific steps you can take to improve your body's ability to eliminate toxins, helping to mitigate the effects of chemical exposures you can't control.

Later on in this book, you'll find a full-body survey that will help you determine your toxin risk, along with a comprehensive 21-Day Plan to help you slash your environmental exposure while boosting your body's ability to detoxify in just three weeks' time. Finally, in the appendices, I tell you which lab tests are worth doing and where to get them done, while also giving you dozens of delicious, detoxifying recipes.

I KNOW THAT many of you reading this right now are concerned about your overall health or you are suffering from symptoms or a condition without any answers—or the right answers, since there's a lot of misinformation online and even in doctor's offices. Some of you may have been told that your symptoms aren't real, that you're not sick, that you just need more rest, or there are no options to treat what you have. Others of you may have been told that your lab work looks "fine," when integrative doctors like me would more likely tell you that what's often considered "normal" or "fine" in conventional medicine doesn't mean optimal or symptom-free. Still others of you may be worried about how to prevent a condition for which you have a family history, or are simply anxious knowing how many toxins exist in our world.

All these concerns are real and valid, and they are the reason I wrote this book: to help you get answers by giving you the tools to do your own detective work; you'll be connecting the dots between your symptoms and the solutions to treat them that are effective, realistic, and sustainable. Most of all, I want to empower you to take control of your body and improve your health—because, no matter who you are, where you live, how much money you make, or your current medical state, you *can* make a big difference in how you feel.

So, buckle up and get ready for an electrifying ride. The journey to a cleaner, healthier you starts when you turn the page.

SECTION I

ASSESS

CHAPTER 1

The Smoking Gun: Environmental Chemicals

THE BATHROOM WAS spinning. Or, I was spinning, standing in the middle of the room, a sea of skincare sprays; bottles of moisturizer, creams, and shampoos; and tiny tubes of makeup and lip gloss, many so colorful that it looked as though someone had upended a candy store on my white-tile floor—except nothing here was sweet or appealing. These were all my personal-care products—cosmetics, creams, shampoos, serums, deodorants, and perfumes—alongside an array of household cleaners I had pulled from other areas of our home, including detergents, disinfectants, air fresheners, insect killers, mold killers, and other all-purpose killers strong enough to annihilate whatever was left. From our kitchen, I had collected cans of soup and tuna, along with boxes of cereal and cookies that may have had enough glyphosate—an herbicide used on wheat and other crops—to earn a place on the ingredients list. There were also things to drink in my pile, including bottles of water, diet sodas, and a jug of cow's milk that had started to sweat through the plastic container.

If this sounds like I was assembling goods for a fallout shelter, you'd be only partially right. But these weren't the products I wanted with me in the unlikely event of an apocalypse. These were the products I was worried would *cause* an apocalypse—not in a far-fetched, end-of-existence, made-for-a-movie kind of way, but in a slow, insidious way, quietly harming my health, the health of my family, and the health of everyone else I knew. That's why I spread out all these products on my bathroom floor: I wanted to know exactly how many chemicals I was exposing my body to on a daily basis. Over time and with more research, I realized I had many more things to add to this pile, including most of my cookware, clothing, electronic devices, furniture, flooring, and other common household items that contain dangerous environmental toxins.

Before I go any further, know that I'm not trying to be dramatic. Professionally, I can't be. For the last twenty-plus years, I've worked as a clinical rheumatologist, which is a doctor who diagnoses and treats inflammatory diseases. In my work with patients, many of whom are critically ill with conditions other doctors don't know how to treat, I've had to remain evidence-based and factual. There's no room for drama when you're trying to help people with crippling conditions for which neither they nor their doctors have any answers. At the same time, I've spent the past two decades reading, researching, and writing about how environmental toxins affect our health. As I've done this, I've also watched this research play out in real time, as the rates of chronic illnesses have climbed steadily among my patients—patients who have been getting diagnosed at younger and younger ages and, most strikingly, without any trace of a family history of their disease.

Let's go back to what was on my bathroom floor. What most people don't realize, including myself at the time, is that more than ninety-five thousand chemicals are currently used in US product markets, and those chemicals are found in everything from our food, water, and personal-care products to our household cleaners, furniture, electronics, toys, construction materials, and more.[1] In short, if something is manufactured in our modern age, it probably contains at least one synthetic chemical, if not hundreds. Environmental toxins, including some that were banned decades ago, are also present in the air we breathe, the soil in which we grow our food and from where we source our water, and the oceans, lakes, rivers, and ponds where we swim and fish.

Even though environmental chemicals are allowed to be used, many have been indisputably linked to serious health conditions, including cancer, heart disease, diabetes, obesity, neurological disorders like Alzheimer's disease, and autoimmune diseases like rheumatoid arthritis. Environmental toxins are also associated with troubling ailments like chronic pain, fatigue, weight gain, hair loss, gastrointestinal troubles, and premature aging.[2] What's more, the majority of the chemicals used today—we're talking tens of thousands of toxins—have *never* been tested for human safety. Like never.[3] As in, no safety testing *ever*. And if past history is any indicator of future outcomes, many chemicals may be problematic if they were to be tested, given the results of those toxins that have already been analyzed.

In my thirties, after I took stock of my daily chemical exposure in that bathroom, I started making small tweaks to my diet and lifestyle. Not big, sweeping, move-off-the-grid changes but simple, sustainable adjustments to my routine that could lower my risk of what are known as *diseases of civilization*—conditions like cancer, heart disease, and obesity that are largely preventable by lifestyle change. Since then, I've done a pretty good job at reining in the toxins I *can* control. I also recognize that no one can ever be perfect, and that my journey, like that of anyone else's, is ongoing.

I haven't made every change possible. I still dye my hair (chemical-free hair color just doesn't do it for me) and occasionally I eat foods with problematic toxins, since it's difficult to avoid all chemicals in all foods.

While I examine almost everything I buy, I've learned how to be time-efficient about it while also saving money. I won't lie: eating mostly organic foods and buying chemical-free consumer products can be expensive, so I've come up with some hacks and tips to save money while making safer choices (which I share throughout this book).

This result reflects my overall ethos: *limiting your exposure to environmental toxins is about making smart, strategic choices, not grave sacrifices or break-the-bank purchases.* The truth is, you can't avoid all environmental toxins—it just isn't possible. You also can't live in fear. Instead, I want to empower you to take control of your health so you can increase your chances of not only living longer but also living better.

What It Means to Be "Healthy": My Journey from Unnecessary Exposure to Better Well-Being

Before my dog Truxton died in 2008, igniting my personal investigation into environmental chemicals, I considered myself to be fairly healthy. I jogged a few times a week, brought salads to work so I wouldn't be tempted by the carb-heavy catering sponsored by pharmaceutical companies, and slathered on sunscreen before I stepped outside every morning. Sure, I had a thing for Oreos and I loved to squirt Cheez Whiz out of the can, but who doesn't have their indulgences? I figured that as long as my weight was within a healthy range, then it was no harm, no foul.

I also considered myself somewhat proactive about environmental toxins, especially after my husband and I moved from New York City to a small farming town outside Princeton, New Jersey. Our new home—actually an old barn we renovated—backed up onto acres of corn, soy, and potato fields. What we didn't know is that for years those fields had been sprayed with harsh agricultural chemicals. From neighbors,

I heard horror stories about how, only a few decades earlier, planes would swoop down and soak the fields with pesticides, even as children and pets played nearby. The aftermath would be visible, leaving a dusty residue on window screens, doors, backyard playgrounds, and any toys left outside by little hands.

While we drank the tap water in New York City without hesitation (didn't New York have the best water for making bagels, after all?), my husband and I began buying bottled water when we moved to New Jersey because we were worried that the town's groundwater supply had been contaminated with pesticides. Lugging plastic water bottles home by the case from the supermarket, I felt proud of myself for what seemed, at the time, like taking a preventative measure for my health and the health of my family. After several months, though, we ditched the store-bought bottles in favor of home water filters, not because we believed them to be any healthier but because we realized they'd be more convenient.

Shortly after we moved to New Jersey, I became pregnant with my first son. I immediately stopped drinking alcohol and cut out raw fish and cold cuts, the latter two carrying a risk of infection for pregnant women.[4] But I was also ravenous all the time. I started stopping at McDonald's to get their signature Big Breakfast with Hotcakes. The meal, served piping hot in a plastic to-go container, came with scrambled eggs, hash browns, sausage, biscuits, and hotcakes (which I perceived to be pancakes), complete with artificially flavored maple syrup and orange juice. I usually wolfed down the breakfast while in my car on my way to work, eating out of the plastic container using the plastic utensils they gave me. I did this while reconciling all the calories and saturated fat I was consuming—what I thought were the unhealthiest components of the meal at the time—with the fact I needed the fuel for a growing baby boy.

My addiction to the Big Breakfast grew so acute that, immediately after I gave birth, I was ready to shout obscenities at the hospital staff if I couldn't get my hands on those hotcakes. My husband, aware of my cravings, good-heartedly drove to a nearby diner to pick up some for me and snuck the greasy goods into the maternity ward.

Two years after our first son was born, I got pregnant again and gave birth to another boy. As our family grew, so did my measures to keep our kids and home safe and healthy. This meant constantly cleaning the house to protect the two young boys from the dirt, dust, and possible pathogens you might expect to find in an old barn. I was proud of our "new" home—it was the first one I had owned outside of city apartments—and I wanted it to look and be as comfortable as possible. I Windexed the windows until they were streak-free, mopped the floors with Mr. Clean until I could smell the pine-lemon scent from another room, and bleached every surface of our bathrooms on a regular basis. I used wasp spray, ant spray, and termite spray inside the house and regularly doused our dog and cat in flea and tick sprays to prevent Lyme disease, a serious concern for rheumatologists like me. Usually, I'd wash my hands after handling these products, although probably not all the time and probably not thoroughly. After all, I was busy, busy, busy, building a new medical practice, starting a new family, and creating a new home. And I trusted that everything I was using was safe, or else it wouldn't be sold in stores.

Living in a house also introduced me to a wide new world of consumer goods. I became obsessed with air fresheners, for example, and quickly amassed a drawerful, with scents like ocean breeze, strawberry fields, and pumpkin spice that promised to turn our home into a California vacation spot or a rustic country bakery. At any given time, especially in the fall and during the holidays, I had two perfumed plug-ins gently pumping away, delivering an olfactory symphony of peppermint and cinnamon into the air.

I was also a sucker for the heavily scented shampoos and conditioners so popular at the time—the "fruitier" the scent, the better. And while I didn't wear a ton of makeup—lip gloss, eye shadow, and mascara at most, with some eyeliner and concealer if I was feeling fancy—I still managed to collect an immense (perhaps embarrassing) supply of free samples from cosmetic companies.

But after Truxton died, I realized I had been ingesting, absorbing, inhaling, or otherwise exposing myself to hundreds of chemicals every day. Every perfumed product, like my air fresheners and scented hair products, was rife with synthetic "fragrance," which can contain more than three thousand undisclosed ingredients and chemicals in a single term.[5] The undisclosed chemicals in the word *fragrance* or *perfume* usually contain phthalates, a large class of chemicals that have been shown to disrupt normal hormone function, immune system function, and genitalia development in newborn male babies. Phthalates have also been found to increase the risk of thyroid and other hormone-sensitive cancers, among other serious health concerns.[6] Parabens, another class of chemicals found in personal-care products and my little "freebie" samples on the bathroom floor, have been linked to breast cancer[7] and even found in breast-tissue samples from both benign and cancerous breasts.[8] Many of my personal-care products also contained pegylated chemicals, which are purposefully designed to permeate the protective layers of skin, carrying other chemicals straight into the bloodstream. There were hundreds of other chemicals in the products on my bathroom floor, too, many of which you'll read about in the pages that follow. Suddenly, I was overwhelmed. And I was ready for a change.

Today, I'm no longer overwhelmed. I'm informed. I'm thankful that I've learned how to live a healthier life and can now impart that wisdom to others. Every day is another chance to learn, too, as new research is published and new solutions are shared. Lowering your chemical exposure is a journey, not a destination.

Through it all, I can say one thing with certainty: No matter who you are, the lifestyle you lead, or how many points of exposure you believe may be unavoidable, *there are simple, sustainable steps you can take to reduce your toxic load and lower your overall disease risk.* Eliminating just a few toxins from your daily life can have a significant impact on your physical health and overall well-being. What's more, adopting certain lifestyle habits can go a long way toward protecting your body against the chemical exposure that you do incur.

How do I know this? The existing levels of many common chemicals can be detected in tests of bodily fluids, like urine, blood, breast milk, and breast tissue. When we make changes to reduce our exposure to these chemicals, the levels of those chemicals in our bodily fluids drop, too, reducing our risk of developing diseases now associated with those chemicals.

In other words, the future is yours: *All you have to do is begin the journey.*

The Truth About Environmental Chemicals and Your Health

I believe that environmental chemicals are the number one cause of most acute and chronic health conditions. In fact, some studies even show that 90 percent of all illnesses are environmentally associated, stemming primarily from smoking, alcohol, and air pollution,[9] in addition to consuming processed foods.[10] At the very least, the World Health Organization estimates that one in four deaths worldwide is due to unhealthy environments where people are exposed to an excess of synthetic chemicals; pollutants in air, water, and/or soil; and/or other environmental risk factors.[11]

I'm not sharing these statistics with you to stir alarm. Instead, I want to demonstrate that you *do* have agency over the future of your health. While not all environmental chemicals are avoidable, many are, so taking proactive steps now—no matter how much exposure you've incurred—can significantly reduce your risk of developing both acute and chronic conditions.

What exactly are acute and chronic health conditions? *Acute health conditions* develop suddenly, generally last a short period of time, and include illnesses like asthma attacks, respiratory infections, food allergy reactions, and rashes or dermatitis. *Chronic health conditions*, on the other hand, tend to build up over a longer period of time and are often caused by lifestyle habits, such as an unhealthy diet, chronic psychological stress, cigarette smoking, and physical inactivity—which is why they're called "lifestyle diseases" or, as I noted earlier in this chapter, "diseases of civilization."[12] Examples of chronic health conditions include cancer, heart disease, dementia, diabetes, obesity, depression, and autoimmune diseases.

How can environmental chemicals be the primary cause of such a wide array of medical conditions? As you're learning, environmental toxins are everywhere, including in the food we eat, the water we drink, and the personal-care products and cleaning supplies we use. They're also found in our electronics, clothing, cookware, cars, furniture, flooring, and building materials, as well as in the lawns, athletic fields, forests, backyards, and beaches where we and our children play. In short, most places and most consumer products have environmental toxins, even if we can't see or smell them—or there's no label or warning sign alerting us to their presence.

One reason environmental chemicals are so influential in disease risk is that they can be toxic in very small amounts. Many chemicals, including bisphenol A (BPA), are used to make food and beverage containers, while phthalates are found in everything from personal-care products to medical devices. Both may be just as, if not more, harmful in low doses[13] than in large amounts because of a phenomenon known as *non-monotonic dose response*. This phenomenon, which goes against predictable dose patterns, produces toxic effects at low doses similar to the way hormones in infinitesimal amounts can have enormous physiological effects.[14] In these instances, the dose does *not* make the poison. This is troubling, given that up to 99 percent of the population has detectable levels of BPA in their blood, sweat, or urine,[15] while most of us also have measurable levels of phthalate metabolites.[16]

It's also not just what one chemical in your moisturizer, mascara, yoga pants, or diet soda is doing to your health—it's what all these chemicals in combination might do, which is an unknown X factor that is nearly impossible to test or control for. If you ever took high-school chemistry, you know that chemicals can interact with each other, sometimes in significant or unpredictable ways. Today, we're doing the same thing with our bodies, conducting a crude science experiment by exposing ourselves to different chemical cocktails for which neither we nor scientists can predict the consequences. The outcome may also be more serious than what we might think, as we expose our bodies to chemical mixtures that may compound or synergize the harmful effects that individual toxins pose on their own.

Environmental chemicals are such an intrinsic part of our everyday, modern lives that scientists recently coined the term *exposome* to describe what we now face: chemical exposure from the day we're conceived in the womb until the day we die. The exposome (not to be confused with the body's *microbiome*, which is an entirely different concept) describes all the environmental exposures we have through life, which include what we eat, how high or low our stress levels are, which drugs we take, and the levels of pollution we face, and how these varying exposures affect our health. Through the lens of our exposome, researchers now know that environmental chemicals can affect our DNA, modifying activity in real time by turning on or off certain genes.[17] This phenomenon is known as *epigenetics*, which is the ability of factors in our environment and personal behaviors to alter our gene expression over our lifetime. While diet, body mass index, tobacco consumption, physical activity, and psychological stress all play a role in epigenetics, one of the most influential factors is our exposure to environmental chemicals.

The good news about epigenetics, however, is that we also know which lifestyle factors can positively impact our gene activity. These factors include eating a nutritionally dense diet, moving our bodies in more regular and meaningful ways, and lowering psychological stress, among other habits covered in later chapters. So, while we may not be able to entirely obviate the impact of all environmental toxins on our gene activity, we can certainly adopt new habits to counteract their negative effects. Throughout this book, I share with you some targeted ways to influence your genes in real time and to effectively hack your exposome.

The Missing Link: Environmental Chemicals, Immune Health, and Inflammation

If you want to reduce your chemical exposure in targeted, effective ways, it pays to know how environmental toxins affect the body on a biological level. Once you understand the biology of the problem, you can determine what you need to do to remedy it. Or, as former Apple CEO Steve Jobs is credited with saying, "If you define the problem correctly, you almost have the solution."[18] So, let's define the problem.

Environmental chemicals are harmful to our health because they interfere with the normal function of nearly every system in the body, including our respiratory, cardiovascular, reproductive, nervous, and endocrine systems. This is not a reason to freak out, however; we've been living among environmental chemicals for years and will be for years more, similar to how we live with harmful viruses and bugs. Instead, it's a reason to keep reading. Like avoiding the common cold and flu, there are things you can do to avoid environmental chemicals once you know what they are.

To date, most of the research on environmental chemicals and human health has focused on the endocrine system, which is a network of glands that work together to monitor, manufacture, and regulate hormones throughout the body (think the thyroid hormone for metabolism; insulin to help manage blood glucose; sex hormones for fetal development, growth, and fertility; and adrenal gland hormones to help control blood pressure). In short, the hormones controlled by our endocrine system affect nearly every one of our physical processes, including our metabolism, mood, fertility, growth and development, sexual function, and sleep.

Environmental toxins can disrupt normal endocrine function in different ways.[19] Some endocrine-disrupting chemicals (EDCs) disrupt the normal production of hormones, including estrogen, testosterone, insulin, thyroid hormone, and growth hormone. EDCs can also mimic hormones, fooling the organs and body into either under- or over-responding with less or more hormones, which can result in hyper- or hypothyroidism, diabetes, and hypertension. Some EDCs increase cell growth in tissues. Others affect the type of cells made by bone marrow (stem cells), misdirecting them to become fat cells instead of platelets or immune cells.

Common EDCs include bisphenol A (BPA), phthalates, triclosan (found in cooking utensils and personal-care products), polychlorinated biphenyls (PCBs, which were banned decades ago but because they persist for a long time, they still contaminate some fish, meat, and dairy products), and per- and polyfluoroalkyl substances (PFAS, known as the "forever chemicals," which are found in a plethora of items like cleaning supplies, nonstick cookware, stain- and water-resistant fabric, dental floss, fire extinguishers, and personal-care products).[20] That's a lot of acronyms for chemicals in common products, but again, there's no need to freak out: you'll learn in this book how to avoid them to the best of your ability.

Because of their ability to disrupt hormone function, EDCs have been linked to hormone-sensitive cancers (for example, breast, testicular, thyroid, endometrial, uterine), diabetes, heart problems, respiratory ailments, metabolic complications, altered nervous system function, endometriosis, lowered fertility, neurological disorders, and a host of other health conditions.[21] In 2012, the World Health Organization declared EDCs a "global threat that should be addressed,"[22] prompting a frenzy of research on that class of chemicals. And you can feel good that you're addressing the problem personally: you picked up this book!

Unfortunately, environmental toxins don't just affect our endocrine system, though. They also interfere with our immune system, which is our body's best and only defense against disease. In fact, most common EDCs are also IDCs, or *immune-disrupting chemicals*, which are environmental toxins that interfere with the normal function of our immune system. Like EDCs, IDCs have been linked to cancer, diabetes, heart disease, autoimmune diseases, neurological diseases, obesity, asthma, allergies, weight gain, premature aging, an increased susceptibility to infectious diseases, and a blunted response to vaccines, among many other ailments.

The impact of today's environmental toxins on our immune health is a big reason why I wrote this book. As a rheumatologist, I know from my medical training and clinical experience that the strength of our immune system matters immensely for our overall health and well-being. Without a strong immune system, we get sick. And one reason we get sick is that there is a process our immune system directly governs—namely, our degree of internal inflammation.

Over the past few decades, *inflammation* has become a buzzword among health experts and influencers—and for good reason.

Inflammation is our immune system's natural response to injury, infection, or foreign substances that enter our bodies and that our immune cells don't recognize. When our immune system is confronted with one of these factors, it sends out an army of inflammatory cells to help heal, fight off, or neutralize the problem.

There are two types of inflammation: acute and chronic. *Acute inflammation* happens when we incur a sudden injury or infection, such as if we were to cut a finger, break a bone, get stung by a bee, or become exposed to a virus like a cold or the flu. With acute inflammation, we experience immediate symptoms that include pain, redness, and swelling, and these symptoms eventually subside in a matter of hours, days, or weeks.

Chronic inflammation, on the other hand, occurs when our immune system is continually triggered by a foreign substance, causing it to produce an inflammatory response over and over again. While we can't always see or touch chronic inflammation, it can result in symptoms that include fatigue, weight gain, gastrointestinal complications, chronic pain, skin rashes, and depression, anxiety, and other mood disorders. Over time, if left untreated, chronic inflammation can lead to cancer, heart disease, diabetes, neurodegenerative diseases like Alzheimer's, and autoimmune diseases, the last of which occur when the immune system attacks its own healthy tissue.[23] Illnesses caused by chronic inflammation now contribute to more than half of all deaths worldwide, according to global estimates.[24]

One of the leading causes of chronic inflammation is environmental toxins.[25] Every time we're exposed to an immune-disrupting chemical, our body perceives the substance to be an invader and launches an inflammatory attack on it. Since we're all exposed to hundreds of IDCs every day—no matter our age, race, income bracket, or country of residence—our immune system keeps activating an inflammatory response, creating a state of chronic inflammation. As a result, most of us suffer from chronic inflammation to some degree. And unfortunately, that chronic inflammation is making many of us sick.

Why doesn't our immune system adapt to IDCs like it does to some viruses, bacteria, and other invaders that we're routinely exposed to during our lifetime? The short answer is that our immune system hasn't had enough time to evolve—or more specifically, the part of our immune system known as our *adaptive immune system* hasn't had enough time to evolve.[26] You see, our immune system is an ancient and exquisite system that has protected humans from outside invaders for millennia. But over the last century or so, our immune system has rapidly been introduced to hundreds of new synthetic chemicals or attackers against which it's had no time to evolve responses. Let's take a closer look at this.

Our immune system is made up of two parts: our *innate immune system*, or the one we were born with that's been "hardwired" over millions of years of human evolution to recognize invaders; and our *adaptive immune system*, which can change during our lifetime to combat new substances we've never encountered before. Covid-19 is a great example of how our adaptive immune system works. While Covid-19 was a "new" virus, our adaptive immune system was able to create antibodies to fight it off when we were first exposed to the illness, whether through a vaccine or infection. What helped our immune system create those antibodies is that Covid-19 is not so dissimilar from what our body has seen in our evolutionary past. First, it's a natural virus; and second, it belongs to a family of coronaviruses that researchers estimate has existed among human beings for centuries.[27]

Most man-made chemicals, on the other hand, have existed for less than a hundred years or so, ever since the start of industrial chemical manufacturing and mostly following World War II. From the perspective of our immune system, a hundred years isn't even a blip on the metaphorical radar screen of human evolution. What's more, because environmental chemicals are synthetic (meaning "not natural"), and generally incredibly potent, they are more "foreign" to our immune system than those natural invaders. For these reasons, environmental chemicals have been shown to interfere with the body's synthesis of cytokines, or immune proteins that help control inflammation, and immunoglobins, a type of antibody.[28] Some chemicals, like BPA, which is found in canned foods and thermal ink paper (for example, receipts or boarding passes), may be broken down by the human body in just a few hours—although because billions of pounds of BPA are used in so many products, virtually everyone, everywhere is continuously exposed to it.[29] However, other chemicals may take months or even years to be cleared by the body—and the longer they stick around, the more potential risk for health issues. This is especially true of "forever chemicals" like the perfluoroalkyl substances known as PFAS, which are found in nonstick cookware, food packaging, drinking water, and dozens of other products. They're called "forever chemicals" because they don't break down over time. (You'll learn much more about PFAS and how to avoid them in the chapters that follow.) These dangerous toxins may suppress our immune system's ability to combat infection and reduce the efficacy of some vaccines by blunting the intended antibody response, according to the research.[30]

Understanding how environmental toxins affect our immune system thus gives us an incredible opportunity to fight back. When we know why and how the IDCs affect our bodies, we also can know what to do about it: we can take steps to *bolster the strength of our immunity and lower our levels of chronic inflammation*. (Further along in this book, I share with you exactly how to do both.)

The fact that these chemicals are allowed to exist in our environment is infuriating, and it's okay to be angry and scared. But you don't have to live in fear anymore. In this book, I'll help you make the best lifestyle changes you can so as to lower your exposure—changes that make sense for you and your loved ones. And these lifestyle changes do work. Today, when I test my blood for the existence of environmental chemicals, my results are incredible. For example, while 97 percent of Americans have detectable levels of PFAS in their blood, I don't.[31] My levels of urinary BPA, one of the most pervasive chemicals worldwide, have also dropped dramatically. And it's not just me; study after study shows that making lifestyle changes to lower your exposure to the chemicals found in water, food, cosmetics and other personal-care products, and home goods do work, and can significantly reduce your risk of disease and the adverse health effects caused by environmental toxins. In other words, small changes really do work and will reduce risk.

Chapter 1 Takeaways

- More than ninety-five thousand synthetic chemicals are "approved" for use in the United States, but only a small percentage have been tested by regulatory agencies for any general health effects and hardly any for specific IDC effects.
- Most of us are exposed to hundreds, if not thousands, of chemicals every day in our air, food, water, personal-care products, electronics, homes, and offices.
- Synthetic chemicals interfere with the normal function of our body's major systems, including our nervous, respiratory, cardiovascular, reproductive, endocrine, and immune systems. A major way that synthetic chemicals harm our health is by constantly creating inflammation in the body, which over time can lead to chronic illnesses like cancer, heart disease, diabetes, Alzheimer's disease, and other neurological disorders, and autoimmune diseases.
- Small changes to your lifestyle can make a huge difference to your risk of developing disease.

CHAPTER 2

Your Body on Chemicals

ASHLEY COULDN'T STOP staring at her hands. Swollen and slightly twisted, her fingers looked more like "deformed sausages," as she described them, than what you'd expect to see in a relatively healthy twenty-seven-year-old woman. She held her hands out as she greeted me, then pulled them back to unfasten her coat, struggling and wincing as she pushed the buttons through the holes. I helped her with her jacket, then we looked at her hands together, as she sat on the edge of my medical exam table. I asked if she had difficulty doing any other tasks, and she said her hands were often so swollen and painful that she couldn't cut up food for her one-year-old son, or even grip his little hand at times. Her fingers looked so gnarled now, she added, that she worried everyone was staring at her when she pushed a cart through the grocery store or picked up her son at the playground. I empathized. Disease is never easy, but when you feel as though you're all alone or are abnormal, that emotional suffering can make the physical discomfort that much more acute.

As I continued with the exam, I asked Ashley to take off her shoes. Immediately, I could see that her toes were swollen as well, which she said she assumed was a normal, long-term side effect of pregnancy. I assured her that it wasn't, and I asked if she ever felt stiff in the morning. She did, although the tension usually went away after a few hours. Still, she was constantly tired, she said, despite getting at least eight hours' sleep each night. She wondered if she had failed somehow to adjust to new motherhood. But chronic fatigue is never anyone's fault or something a person has to put up with, I told her, no matter how busy or how stressful their lives might be.

From the looks of her swollen finger and toe joints, Ashley clearly had arthritis, which is defined as inflammation, pain, and/or stiffness in the joints. The trick was to identify *which* kind of arthritis, as there are more than a hundred types. Arthritis can be due to an infection like Lyme disease, a medical condition like gout, or a musculoskeletal problem like osteoarthritis. But after listening to her symptoms and doing a full intake, I had a pretty good idea what Ashley might be suffering from. Like so many people, especially younger and younger women, Ashley appeared to have rheumatoid arthritis (RA), an autoimmune disease marked by joint pain, swelling, and inflammation that can affect anyone at any age.

Autoimmune diseases like RA occur when the body's immune system attacks healthy tissue along with the harmful cells. This situation has historically been blamed on a confluence of factors that have included genetics and environmental exposure. Today, however, many researchers believe that the United States's skyrocketing rates of autoimmune disease in the last thirty years is due to the country's concurrent skyrocketing rates of chemical exposure.[1] Compounding the problem is that many patients like Ashley, who had no family history of autoimmunity, often see a handful of doctors before being properly diagnosed, as there's no "standard of care" for autoimmune diseases—meaning there's no universally accepted medical method to identify and treat the broad spectrum of immune conditions, many of which do not meet the full criteria for established or "classic" autoimmune disease classification.

More often than not, autoimmune diseases may present as a variety of symptoms that appear to be separate ailments—but they aren't. While they can be the result of anything from infection and physical trauma to simply too much stress, they can also be triggered or exacerbated by environmental exposure. What's more, women are, in general, twice as likely to be diagnosed with autoimmune diseases as men, as I explain on page 39.[2]

In Ashley's case, I first wanted to order blood tests that would show rheumatoid markers, in addition to markers that might reveal a thyroid problem, nutritional deficiencies, infection, and/or a family history of RA (through genetic testing). I also wanted to hear her *whole* health story (not just a list of her past surgeries and current medications), including what she regularly ate, what kind of water she drank (tap, filtered, or bottled?), how long and how frequently she exercised, how she managed her stress, which prescription drugs she was taking and had taken in the past, and what her childhood had been like. For example, did she grow up in a city or near a farm or industrial plant? What kind of illnesses had she had as a kid and did she frequently take antibiotics? Did she grow up in a family that ate home-cooked meals or did she consume mostly highly processed foods? Had she grown up in a stressful home and/or experienced childhood trauma, or did she have a mostly emotionally supportive and physically active childhood? What types of diseases ran in her family?

This is what integrative medicine is all about. Integrative physicians consider the whole person, not just the isolated body part or system impacted by disease. We look at a patient's daily habits, like diet, exercise, and toxin exposure, because we know that most diseases are influenced by, if not the result of, these lifestyle factors. If you think of your body like a car, for instance, integrative doctors want to make sure you're not filling the tank with the wrong grade of gasoline, or not starting it up for weeks at a time, or not leaving it outside in the rain for days. All habits, including diet, activity level, and toxin exposure, can create problems for any machine.

I asked Ashley these questions, in addition to a few others. Her answers gave me a ton of insight into what might be happening within this young woman's body. And from what she told me, it was clear that Ashley's microbiome—the vast collection of bacteria, fungi, yeast, viruses, and other microorganisms that live in the body—had taken multiple "hits," as I like to call them. As a child, Ashley had suffered from frequent strep throat and ear infections, and as a result, she had taken multiple courses of antibiotics at an early age. While these drugs can be lifesaving and are often necessary at times, antibiotics also kill off the microbiome's "good" bacteria in addition to the bad stuff. That's a problem for many reasons, including that good bacteria help metabolize those environmental toxins and actually prevent them from entering the bloodstream. What's more, when young children take antibiotics, doing so can interfere with the development and ultimate composition of their gut microbiome, increasing the risk of illness later in life.[3]

Another hit was Ashley's diet. As a kid, she lived on frozen meals, cereal, and sandwiches, all which can contain food and food-packaging chemicals now capable of being detected in human blood, breast milk, and urine. While she had "cleaned up" her diet after college, prioritizing "healthy" choices like plant-based protein shakes, veggie burgers, and seltzer instead of sugar-free soda, these items can unfortunately still be rife with toxins. Many protein powders, for example, contain bisphenol A (BPA), a chemical known to affect hormone and immune function. BPA can also be found in canned foods, thermal-ink receipts, and some food packaging, in addition to pesticides and heavy metals like lead and cadmium. (Research also suggests these contaminants may be higher in plant-based protein powders than powders made from dairy and egg).[4] Likewise, veggie burgers, along with other plant-based meat alternatives, can contain elevated levels of synthetic preservatives and food dyes.[5] And cans of seltzer (as opposed to those sold in glass bottles), including many flavored varieties that have become increasingly popular in recent years, can include BPA—or just-as-harmful BPA analogs like bisphenol S (BPS) or bisphenol F (BPF).[6]

If any of these items are a regular part of your diet, not to worry—in fact, I'd give yourself a little pat on the back, since these products in themselves aren't necessarily unhealthy. What makes them possibly detrimental to our microbiome is how the food manufacturers grow the ingredients, process the products, or package them. As we'll discuss in chapter 8, reducing your toxin exposure isn't necessarily about changing your habits so much as it is learning to choose those products or types of packaging that contain fewer known toxins.

Since Ashley had taken multiple courses of antibiotics at a critical age and had consumed foods high in chemical additives for so many years, I suspected she might have gut dysbiosis, a common condition in which someone has an imbalance of microorganisms in their intestinal tract, with more bad microbes than good ones.[7] If she did have dysbiosis, it might explain her RA, since the condition is one of the leading causes of autoimmune conditions, according to the research.[8] Gut dysbiosis can also lead to other chronic illnesses like cancer, diabetes, obesity, infertility, and neurodegenerative disorders like Alzheimer's.[9]

How can an imbalance of bacteria do all this? In short, the gut microbiome is the center of gravity for our entire immune system, supporting and anchoring the majority of our body's immune activity. And anything that shifts our gut microorganisms in one way will ultimately shift our immunity in a corresponding way.

After hearing Ashley's health story, I recommended we also do a stool analysis, in addition to tests for RA. A stool analysis is a series of tests that can show the kinds of microbes living in the intestinal tract and can indicate a diagnosis of gut dysbiosis. Although the makeup of our poop is ever changing and varies from meal to meal, the results of her stool analysis would open up a discussion on reasonable dietary improvement. Several weeks later, we had the results: Ashley had both RA and gut dysbiosis. When she came into my office again, I told her we'd have to treat both if she wanted to begin to resolve her symptoms. While prescription drugs would certainly help, drugs alone wouldn't solve her autoimmune condition if it was triggered or fueled by gut dysbiosis—we needed to go "upstream" to find the root cause of her immune illness. Ashley would have to heal her microbiome if she wanted to effectively treat her RA, cleaning up the ecosystem in her gut. And doing this, first and foremost, meant reducing her consistent exposure to environmental chemicals.

IN THIS CHAPTER, we look at how the health of our microbiome is directly and profoundly impacted by the environmental toxins we ingest, and why and how it can lead to symptoms and disease. We also explore how many chemicals can affect our metabolism, making it nearly impossible to lose or maintain weight, no matter what we eat. Finally, we examine how toxins can affect our brain through what's known as the *gut-brain axis*, leading to mood changes, headaches or migraines, and an increased risk of depression, anxiety, and neurological disorders.

While it can be alarming to learn the ways in which environmental chemicals affect different areas of your body, when you understand the pathways that drive illness and disease, you can also see ways to prevent possible symptoms and sickness. So, let's get started.

WHY WOMEN ARE MORE LIKELY TO BE DIAGNOSED WITH AUTOIMMUNE DISEASES

Women are much more likely than men to be affected by autoimmune diseases, a category of illness that includes more than a hundred conditions, such as rheumatoid arthritis, systemic lupus erythematosus (the most common type of lupus), psoriasis, multiple sclerosis, Crohn's disease, and Sjogren's syndrome, the last of which is a condition characterized by dry eyes and dry mouth as a result of the immune system's attacking the glands that make tears, saliva, and moisture for other areas of the body.[10] In fact, autoimmune conditions are so common among women that approximately 80 percent of all people diagnosed with an autoimmune disease are female.

While researchers aren't entirely sure why this is, one of the most supported theories is that estrogens (female sex hormones) stimulate an immune response to immune cells, whereas androgens (male sex hormones) have the exact opposite effect.[11] In other words, the estrogens in a woman's body may overstimulate immune activity—which is why autoimmune conditions are more common in women ages twenty to forty-five, a period when their bodies make more estrogen.

Researchers also believe that sex hormones affect the type and diversity of microorganisms in the gut microbiome, leading to sex-dependent changes in immunity, gastrointestinal inflammation, and susceptibility to inflammatory and immune diseases.[12] Other research suggests women may suffer from more autoimmune diseases owing to a type of faulty RNA protein related to the X chromosome, also known as the Xist gene.[13] Finally, all the

EDCs and IDCs found in our air, food, drinking water, and personal-care and cleaning products can mimic estrogen, thereby increasing total estrogen activity and immune response.[14]

The take-home here is this: If you're female and suspect you may have an autoimmune disease, use this science to make sure you get the tests and answers you need. Unfortunately, many healthcare practitioners may still overlook autoimmune conditions or even dismiss the possibility. You may need to see a doctor who specializes in autoimmune conditions, such as a rheumatologist.

Environmental Toxins and Your Microbiomes

The microbiome isn't just in your stomach. You have microbiomes all over your body, including in your gut, mouth, skin, lungs, nose, belly button, vagina, and/or around your genitals. These massive microbiomes are made up of trillions of different kinds of bacteria, viruses, yeasts, fungi, and other types of microorganisms. In fact, you have more microbial cells and genes in and on your body than you do human cells and genes—to the extent that you're only 43 percent "human," according to researchers.[15] But of all the microbiomes in your body, the microbes in your gut are the biggest and most influential, accounting for three to five pounds of total body weight.

Your gut microbiome is also the main way environmental toxins get into the body, according to scientific studies.[16] What this means is that the chemicals you ingest through your food and drink, and how they affect your gut microbiome, pose the biggest risk to your overall health.

Your gastrointestinal tract, which houses your gut microbiome, is approximately twenty-four feet long, with a surface area of more than four thousand square feet—equivalent to about two tennis courts. Despite your gastrointestinal tract's incredible size, its interior lining—or what separates your interior gut wall from the food moving through your body—is only about half the width of a strand of human hair. These dimensions make your gut both extremely absorbent and extremely vulnerable, as one of the largest interfaces in the body between your outside world and your inner existence.[17]

The microorganisms inside your gut serve many critical purposes, including maintaining the structural integrity of your gastrointestinal tract's paper-thin lining. But if you develop gut dysbiosis, as Ashley had, it can lead to a condition known as *leaky gut*, which occurs when the gut lining becomes compromised or inflamed, allowing food, toxins, bacterial by-products, and other substances to enter the bloodstream, where they can cause inflammation and increase the disease risk. Symptoms of leaky gut often go unnoticed, but when they do manifest, they can include stomach irritability, bloating, increased sensitivity to foods, acid reflux, diarrhea, and/or constipation. Leaky gut, sometimes referred to as *increased intestinal permeability*, can also affect the brain by allowing toxins into the bloodstream that can then cross the delicate blood-brain barrier—stoking neuroinflammation and interfering with healthy neuronal (brain cell) function.[18]

Leaky gut isn't the only possible outcome of an imbalance in gut bacteria. Having gut dysbiosis can also lower your immunity, leading to inflammation, insulin resistance, and oxidative stress, which occurs when your cells have too many free radicals and not enough antioxidants to neutralize them.[19] As mentioned earlier, your gut microbiome is the center of your immune system and hosts up to 80 percent of your total immune cells[20]—that's why gut dysbiosis is often fingered as the "main driver" of immune-based conditions like autoimmune disease, according to the studies.[21]

In particular, gut dysbiosis can prevent your gut microbes from performing critical jobs, like metabolizing the environmental chemicals you do ingest through food and drink.[22] In contrast, a healthy balance of gut flora helps your body digest and absorb nutrients from food and synthesize vitamins,[23] as well as manufacture key enzymes and neurotransmitters like serotonin. In fact, the gut microbiota produce up to 90 percent of your body's total serotonin, which you need for optimal mood, memory, and dozens of other functions (yes, that "feel good" neurotransmitter is made mostly in your gut!).[24] And researchers are just beginning to scratch the surface, finding all the ways a healthy gut can prevent and treat disease and, conversely, how an imbalance may lead to fatigue, weight gain, and premature aging, in addition to more serious symptoms and illness.

What do environmental toxins have to do with your microbiome?

The short answer is: just about everything. As you now know, the toxins you ingest from food and drink can lead to gut dysbiosis and disease.[25] Many of the chemicals mentioned in chapter 1, including BPA, phthalates, PFAS,[26] pesticides, and triclosan (found in personal-care and cleaning products, among other items),[27] have been shown to harm the gut microbiome and cause unhealthy shifts in intestinal flora. Another way to think about this is that if the chemicals sprayed on fruits and vegetables in the growing fields can kill the bugs and other creatures attracted to them, they're also capable of harming the healthy bacteria in your gut.

On the other hand, working to improve your gut health can increase the structural integrity and strength of your gut lining, which can then help prevent toxins from getting into your bloodstream and into your brain. When you have a healthy microbiome, your body is also better able to metabolize the environmental chemicals with which you come in contact. And since your gut microbiome is central to your immunity, bolstering your gut health also bolsters your overall health, limiting the impact those environmental chemicals can have in the first place. For all these reasons, one of the best ways to combat environmental toxins is to support the health of that ecosystem of microbes (your "terrarium," as I tell patients) that thrives within you—and has in all humans for millions of years.

COMMON TOXIC CHEMICALS

CHEMICAL GROUP	FOUND IN	ASSOCIATED HEALTH RISKS
Bisphenols (e.g., BPA, BPS, and similarly structured compounds)	Plastics, canned foods and drinks, water carboys, thermal-ink receipts, dental sealants, IV bags/tubing/respiratory equipment, and other medical equipment	Endocrine effects, immune system effects, autoimmune disease, infertility, thyroid disease, breast cancer
Phthalates (e.g., di-(2-ethylhexyl), dibutyl, di-isodecyl)	Plastics, vinyl flooring, vinyl shower curtains, food storage containers, food packaging, fast food, fragrance/perfumes, lubricating oils, cosmetics and personal care (soaps, shampoos, hair sprays), baby products (lotions), nail polish, bottled water, IV bags/tubing/respiratory equipment, water pipes made from PVC, garden hoses, adhesives, printing inks, insecticides, aspirin, faux leather, carpet tile	Developmental changes in newborns, low birth weight, preterm birth, hormone and immune system effects, autoimmune disease, weight gain, type 2 diabetes, thyroid function, thyroid cancer, increased blood pressure, precocious puberty, semen quality, early menopause, allergies, asthma, delayed neurodevelopment, social impairment
Antimicrobials (e.g., triclosan, Bactroban)	Bar soaps, tile/marble sealant, tampons/feminine-care products, cookware, cleaning products	Immune system effects, hormone disruption, gut microbiome alterations
Flame retardants (e.g., Firemaster 550, polybrominated diphenyl ethers (PBDEs), tetrabromobisphenol A (TBBPA))	Fire extinguishers, uniforms, couches, cables, computer casing	Immune disruption, hormone disruption, cancers, alterations in bone strength, neuroinflammation, neurodegeneration, respiratory problems in newborns

Perfluoroalkyls (PFAS)—"forever chemicals"	Stain protection, water repellent clothing and materials, greaseproof wrappers, nonstick cookware, municipal drinking water, food packaging, carpet/backing, cosmetics, outdoor gear, adhesives/sealants, firefighting foam, car seats	Immune effects, infertility, elevated cholesterol, thyroid disease, reduced vaccine response
Pesticides (e.g., herbicides, insecticides, fungicides)	Used in products to kill weeds, insects, fungus, mold, rodents	Immune effects, neurodegenerative disease, cancers, Parkinson's disease, Celiac disease, autoimmune disease

HEAVY METALS

Lead	Drinking water, water pipes, artificial turf, mining/smelting, paint prior to 1978, smoking	Lowered IQ in children, ADHD, cancers, elevated blood pressure, reproductive dysfunction, kidney disease
Mercury	Fish (especially large fish), shellfish, inhaling mercury vapor or being exposed via skin	Neurotoxicity, Parkinson's disease, immune system disorders, autoimmune disease
Cadmium	Smoking, dark chocolate, drinking water	Cancer, kidney disease, digestive issues, autoimmune disease
Arsenic	Cooked rice, drinking water, some fruit juices, wood preservative, soil, fish and shellfish, smoking	Nausea, skin disorders, several cancers, diabetes, autoimmune disease

Environmental Toxins and Your Metabolism

For those who love to travel, Taylor's job seemed like a dream come true. A pilot for a commercial airline, the fifty-five-year-old had been flying for so long that he could choose his own routes—which is how he frequently ended up in exotic international locations most people experience only in the movies. When overseas, he could spend several days at a time exploring or relaxing in his hotel before flying back home to Newark Airport. That airport is only a little more than an hour's drive from my medical practice in Princeton, New Jersey.

While I marveled at Taylor's foreign adventures, as his physician I knew his job wasn't always ideal, at least not for his health. When we first met several years ago, the pilot was forty pounds overweight, and his mood, ability to move, and overall health were suffering as a result. He'd tried many popular diets, including paleo, keto, and Weight Watchers—sometimes for several months at a time—but nothing seemed to move the needle in a significant or sustainable way.

When Taylor approached me about his weight concerns, I told him that environmental exposure can account for up to 90 percent of a person's total disease risk, which includes conditions like obesity.[28] In other words, environmental chemicals can and do make us fat. If Taylor truly wanted to get to the bottom of his inability to lose weight, he'd have to take a hard look at his chemical exposure and consumption, as well as how to start moving more after those long stints sitting in the cockpit.

The first thing I did as Taylor's doctor was to ask him to take the 50-Question Health and Body Survey (beginning on page 265). When we reviewed his answers together, it was easy to identify at least one major culprit in his chemical exposure: nearly everything he ate and drank came wrapped, boxed, bottled, or canned. This included airplane meals that were heated and served in plastic trays, coffee poured into plastic-lined paper cups, water in plastic bottles, salads packed in plastic or fiber to-go bowls, diet sodas in BPA-lined cans, and sandwiches and other snacks wrapped in greaseproof paper. Adding insult to injury, he regularly consumed these items using plastic cutlery.

While eating and drinking these products on an infrequent basis isn't necessarily going to cause weight gain, Taylor had been ingesting them regularly for the last thirty years—which meant he'd also been ingesting a steady stream of obesogens. Obesogens, which are becoming a hot topic among weight-loss experts, are a class of chemicals shown to disrupt the hormones that directly contribute to weight gain, as well as preventing weight loss through a variety of pathways. Obesogens are a subset of those endocrine-disrupting chemicals (EDCs) that, by definition, increase the white adipose tissue (WAT), or fat cells.[29] While nearly no doctors, dietitians, or diet books emphasize the impact of obesogens on body weight, many scientific researchers would agree that, until Taylor reduced his exposure to these chemicals, it didn't matter what or even how little he ate; he would have a difficult time losing weight.

How can obesogens be so powerful? As EDCs, they interfere with the normal function, activity, or level of the body's hormones, including reproductive, thyroid, growth, blood-sugar regulating (insulin), and hunger-satiating hormones. Disrupting these hormones can be detrimental in many ways, but in regard to weight, they alter the body's delicate dance between energy use and storage—which in turn can stimulate the growth of new fat cells, slow or change the metabolic rate, suppress or activate hormones that control feelings of fullness and hunger, and even cause the body to turn stem cells into fat cells.[30]

Obesogens can also impair the immune system, making them immune-disrupting chemicals (IDCs), as well as EDCs.[31] For anyone trying to lose weight, that's a problem because the immune system may be responsible for up to 40 percent of the body's ability to regulate weight, according to the research.[32] Similarly, obesogens have been shown to cause gut dysbiosis, which directly affects both our immune system and our metabolism.[33] While these effects alone can cause weight gain, gut dysbiosis also lowers the body's ability to neutralize the obesogens to which we are exposed, magnifying their impact on our body mass index and overall health. Finally, obesogens can interfere with how the cells signal one another[34] and disrupt the body's circadian rhythm—the twenty-four-hour internal clock that regulates sleep and stress.[35] The research on obesogens is so damning, in fact, that exposure to this class of chemicals may not only lead to obesity and metabolic problems in us but also in our offspring, editing our epigenome in real time only to get passed along through our sperm and eggs to successive generations.[36]

FOUR COMMON OBESOGENS TO AVOID

At least fifty chemicals are considered to be obesogens, with scientists discovering new toxins with fat-promoting factors every year.[37] Here are some of the most common obesogens:

BISPHENOL A (BPA) AND BPA ANALOGS: Exposure to BPA and its "regrettable substitutes," like bisphenol S (BPS) and bisphenol F (BPF), have been shown to cause weight gain.[38] While banned in plastic baby bottles in the United States and in a handful of other products in certain states, BPA is still "among the highest production-volume chemicals detected in ecosystems, human fluids, and tissues," according to scientists.[39] BPA and its analogs are still found in many plastic beverage bottles and food containers, along with canned foods and sodas, plastic cups and utensils, office watercoolers, kitchen appliances like coffee makers, cash register receipts, boarding passes (BPA acts as a developer for the ink), and personal-care products, among other items. BPA and its analogs are ubiquitous in so many products, in fact, that they're known as "everywhere chemicals."[40]

PHTHALATES: Studies have shown that people exposed to high levels of phthalates are more likely to gain weight.[41] These toxins, also considered to be "everywhere chemicals," are found in a plethora of products, including food packaging, soaps, shampoos, perfumes, shower curtains, toys, and foods via food packaging and processing equipment. Phthalates are one of the most well-studied metabolic disruptors, shown to contribute to insulin resistance and disrupt the production of thyroid hormone and certain sex hormones like testosterone.[42]

TRIBUTYLTIN (TBT): TBT is found in pesticides, disinfectants, and biocides (substances designed to kill living things) and in the paint that coats the bottoms of fishing and shipping vessels. Humans are exposed to TBT through seafood, which absorb the chemical from paint that has leached into the ocean, in addition to foods treated with fungicides or packaged in materials that contain TBT. The chemical can also be found in cleaning products, wood preservatives, and household dust.[43] Today, there's a "considerable body of mechanistic evidence" that TBT is an obesogen, capable of altering metabolism and inducing stem cells to become fat cells.[44] TBT can also break down into dibutyltin (DBT) in the body, where it increases fat tissue and insulin resistance in mice and triggers weight gain in humans.[45] DBT is also found in polyvinyl chloride, a plastic polymer and known endocrine disruptor commonly used to make pipes for public drinking water. This is why filtering your water, as discussed in the next chapter, is so important.

PERFLUOROOCTANOIC ACID (PFOA): One of the class of PFAS "forever chemicals," PFOA is used to make nonstick cookware and microwave popcorn bags, and is found in most public tap water.[46] Owing to its pervasiveness, PFOA is currently detectable in the serum of "nearly all people tested," according to a CDC study.[47] Just recently, the International Agency for Research on Cancer classified PFOA as carcinogenic to humans—the most definitive classification.[48] Exposure to PFOA has been linked with lower resting metabolic rate (how many calories the body burns at rest)[49] and altered insulin production, among other issues.

There are many more known obesogens, and unfortunately the list grows longer every year. The good news, however, is that limiting even some of your exposure can go a long way toward mitigating the effects of obesogens on your weight and overall health.

DO SOMETHING NOW

While you can't avoid BPA and its analogs entirely, you can take steps to reduce your exposure. There is more about ways you can lower your BPA exposure later in the book, but here are some small tips that can make a big difference to your weight-loss efforts and overall health:

- Avoid polycarbonate plastic containers, which are clear and hard, as they are the most likely to contain BPA. To identify them, look for the imprinted triangle with a recycling number 7 or the acronym PC on the bottom of the container.[50] Opt instead for plastics with the number 1, 2, 4, or 5, which usually don't contain BPA.

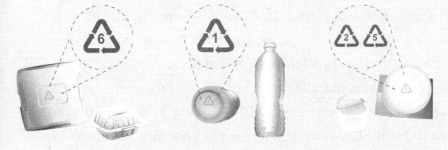

See page 146 for a full list of plastic recycling codes showing specific chemicals in various plastics.

- Never microwave plastic containers or bottles, or put them in the dishwasher, even if they are marked as microwave or dishwasher safe. Also, never leave plastics in a hot car or expose them to heat in any other way.
- Choose fresh or frozen foods over canned goods whenever possible. If you must buy canned products, look for those marked "BPA-free" and rinse the contents vigorously to limit any BPA analogs.
- Ask for receipts to be emailed to you instead of taking a physical copy.

Environmental Toxins and Your Brain

For more than seventeen years, I suffered from crippling migraines. They began shortly after I turned thirteen years old, when suddenly I started to lose part of my vision while experiencing throbbing headaches on one side of my head; they would paralyze me for hours. These headaches would occur two to three times per week, every week, and despite taking prescription migraine medication, nothing seemed to alleviate the frequency or intensity of the headaches.

After I turned thirty and was seeing patients during my hospital residency who had diet-related chronic diseases like obesity, hypertension, and diabetes, I realized that my own diet was terrible and that, even though my weight was within a healthy range, I had to stop eating ultra-processed foods. In a matter of months, my migraines were gone. That was twenty years ago, and in the interim, I can count on one hand how many migraines I've had since.

What had been sparking my migraines, it turns out, was likely the *combination* of toxins I was consuming in those processed foods and in the tap water, in addition to a poor diet that wasn't rich in magnesium, which is essential to preventing and treating migraines. This isn't my speculation as an integrative rheumatologist; rather, it's what studies have shown: low to moderate chemical exposure can trigger migraines.[51] And as it turns out, environmental toxins can increase the risk of mood disorders like depression and anxiety, learning disabilities, memory impairment, autism, ADHD, and decreased IQ in children.[52] Perhaps most alarming, everyday chemicals have been fingered as a primary factor in the development of neurodegenerative diseases like Alzheimer's and Parkinson's.[53]

While environmental chemicals affect the brain through a multitude of pathways, one of the main points of entry is via our gut microbiome and the gut-brain axis. The latter is the unique two-way communication highway between our intestinal microbes and our brain. The vagus nerve, which is the longest cranial nerve in the body, connects our microbiome and brain through a network of small nerve fibers that extend into our gut. These nerve fibers, or fronds, encompass the gut throughout its length and act as a communication highway between the intestinal lining and the brain.[54]

Another way environmental toxins impact the brain is through our immune system, which as you now know is centralized in the gut. When we're exposed to chemicals, our immune system launches an attack on these foreign invaders, which creates inflammation in the body. While acute inflammation is beneficial to helping us handle injury and illness, if our microbiome is constantly bombarded with chemicals and always initiating an inflammatory response, it can lead to chronic neuroinflammation in the brain. Research shows that this kind of neuroinflammation stoked by environmental toxins can lead to depression, cognitive decline, and neurodegenerative disease like Alzheimer's.[55] What's more, the brain has its own immune cells, known as *microglia* and *astrocytes*, which can be impaired by environmental chemicals, undermining our immunity and reducing the integrity of the blood-brain barrier, which helps keep toxins out.[56]

Many environmental toxins have been shown to affect the brain, and many cognitive conditions have a known link to prior chemical exposure. At the same time, many other factors affect the development of cognitive diseases, including age, lifestyle factors, existing illnesses or comorbidities, and gut health, which makes it difficult to pinpoint exactly how much or to what degree certain chemicals cause certain disease. What's more, we all vary in our individual ability to detoxify (something discussed much more in chapter 9) and every environmental exposure is different, depending on the existence of other chemicals alongside a known toxin. For all these reasons, a short exposure to the chemicals might cause illness for some people, while for others, longer exposure would be necessary to trigger symptoms.

That said, here are four cognitive conditions and the environmental chemicals they are associated with, as substantiated by significant research:

- **DEPRESSION AND ANXIETY** have been associated with pesticides; heavy metals like cadmium and lead; air pollution; and secondhand smoke, among other causes.[57]
- **PARKINSON'S DISEASE** has been associated with pesticides, particularly the herbicide paraquat; trichloroethylene, used in dry cleaning and other consumer products and found in groundwater; and polychlorinated biphenyls (PCBs), banned in the United States in 1979 but still existing as a "forever chemical" in food and water, among other causes.[58]
- **ALZHEIMER'S DISEASE** has been associated with heavy metals; pesticides; flame retardants found in consumer goods; and air pollution, among other causes.[59]
- **HEADACHE DISORDERS** have been associated with pesticides; air pollution; preservatives and other additives to processed foods; solvents found in paint and cleaning supplies; and formaldehyde, among other causes.[60]

When It Matters Most: Critical Periods of Exposure

Doing everything you can to reduce your environmental exposure throughout your life can reduce your risk of disease, no matter how old you are or what may be happening inside your body. But there are certain periods of life when we're rapidly developing, or our hormones are more active, and that can cause our immune systems to be more sensitive. During these vulnerable periods, exposure to environmental toxins can have even more deleterious effects. Knowing when those critical periods occur can help you better protect yourself, your children, other family members, and/or other loved ones.

An important note: If you've already had children, don't start to fret about or regret that you may not have done everything possible to limit toxin exposure during pregnancy (or your partner's pregnancy); I hardly knew the advice you'll find in this book when I was pregnant with both my sons. What matters now is taking whatever steps you can to reduce your and your family's exposure. That can go a long way toward limiting the noxious effects that environmental toxins have, no matter your exposure. I certainly wasn't perfect during my pregnancy because I didn't know then. But now that I do know better, I do everything I can to shield my kids from toxic exposure.

Finally, if you have yet to have children, use this information as motivation to do everything you can within your control to protect you (or your partner) from environmental chemicals before becoming (if possible) and while pregnant. Knowledge is power, and as Maya Angelou said, "Do the best you can until you know better. Then when you know better, do better."[61]

PREGNANT WOMEN

You likely already know that what women do during pregnancy can affect a child's future health. It's why pregnant women are advised not to smoke cigarettes, drink alcohol, take recreational drugs, eat sushi or deli meat, or go into hot tubs or saunas, along with other prenatal recommendations. But what's much less widely known is the degree to which exposure to common environmental chemicals during pregnancy can interfere with and alter the development and growth of a fetus's nervous, endocrine, immune, and reproductive systems, increasing the risk of birth defects, cancer, diabetes, obesity, lower IQ, and behavioral problems, among other adverse effects.[62]

One reason pregnancy is such a critical period of exposure is that, contrary to long-held beliefs, the placenta does not serve as a barrier between the chemicals a pregnant woman may be exposed to and those that end up inside a fetus. One older study, for example, found two hundred industrial chemicals in the umbilical-cord blood of newborns, which could potentially raise the risk for developmental conditions or health risks during childhood and into adulthood.[63] More recent research has found industrial chemicals in every organ of every fetus studied, including legacy chemicals like DDT and PCBs, which were banned worldwide decades ago (except for the use of DDT to control malaria in countries outside the United States). But while they were banned, these chemicals are still found in non-organically-managed soil and in ocean water, and they can make their way into the food system.

Another reason pregnancy is such a critical period is that all a child's organ systems develop rapidly during this time, and toxins can interfere with growth, development, and gene expression. This is why alcohol, when consumed by pregnant women, especially during the first trimester when a fetus is rapidly developing, can be so detrimental.

Unfortunately, chemical exposure during pregnancy doesn't just affect a woman and her unborn child: It can also affect that child's children and grandchildren, in a phenomenon known as *multigenerational or transgenerational effects*. A female fetus will develop all her eggs in utero, and males will develop the precursor cell structures for sperm, both of which can be affected by their exposures in the womb.

What to do? If you're pregnant or trying to get pregnant, it's important to take as many of the action steps given in this book as possible to reduce your environmental exposure during this critical time. Trying to reduce your environmental exposure while pregnant is similar to avoiding raw meat, cold cuts, raw seafood, soft cheeses, and the other foods pregnant women are advised to do, since they can contain bacteria that, while a naturally occurring substance, can still raise the risk of fetal harm by causing infection. I advise that pregnant women filter their drinking water using a reverse-osmosis filter (more about this beginning on page 110), eat organic as often as possible, limit consumption of foods packaged in plastic and other synthetic materials, and seriously reduce use of personal-care products made with chemicals. While some points of exposure, like what's in the outdoor air we breathe, are often unavoidable (although there are ways to improve air quality in your home, as outlined in chapter 7), we can control many sources—which is the best and most reassuring truth about our chemical world.

TODDLERS AND YOUNG CHILDREN

During the first seven years of life, a child's brain is developing rapidly, building the basic architecture of the nervous system that will serve for life—it's why an infant can't survive on their own, but a seven-year-old could likely fend for themselves, if necessary. At the same time, a child's reproductive and immune systems grow quickly during the first few years of life, which makes toddlers and young children more vulnerable to endocrine-disrupting chemicals (EDCs) and immune-disrupting chemicals (IDCs) that can alter how these organ systems develop. Exposure to these classes of chemicals, which are found in everything from food and drinking water to furniture, computers, bedding, and soap and other personal-care products (even those formulated for children), may lead to a host of problems, including neurological symptoms like headaches, cognitive development issues, poor growth, DNA damage, thyroid problems, asthma, and other issues.[64]

Pound for pound, toddlers and young children are also more susceptible to chemicals than are larger children and full-grown adults.

They inhale more air per minute; consume proportionally more water, milk, and food; and have a narrower range of food choices. Complicating matters is that young children, with their boundless curiosity and desire to explore, also touch nearly everything they come into contact with, absorbing through their skin or putting into their mouths hands that contain toxic residue found in dust, furniture, and other surfaces, even those that are regularly cleaned (and if you're using conventional chemical cleaners, your young child will be exposed to more toxic residues from these products). Finally, toddlers and young children have immature detoxification systems, reducing their ability to break down individual chemicals, let alone the mixture of chemicals they encounter.[65]

What to do? If you have a toddler or young child at home, it pays to be extra-vigilant about which products you use in the house. Swap out conventional cleaners, air fresheners, and chemical-based laundry detergents for nontoxic supplies, and be vigilant about vacuuming and mopping up dust, which can harbor high levels of toxins released from furniture and other home goods (see chapter 9 for more suggestions). Consider nontoxic linens, mattresses, toys, cribs, car seats, and all other items children may come into contact with, and opt for filtered tap water over giving children bottled water or water that comes straight from the faucet.

Whenever possible and affordable, feed children 100 percent certified organic food (see chapter 8 on how to make this cost-effective), and use only personal-care products that are rated "clean" by a third-party app or website. (I use the Skin Deep database—available online or as a smartphone app called Healthy Living—which is curated by the nonprofit Environmental Working Group [EWG], an entity that rates products on a scale from 1 to 10 based on ingredient toxicity and selects the top choices in every personal-care category.[66] See chapter 6 and the Online Resources appendix for more suggestions.)

If you have toddlers or young children, I also suggest sussing out your childcare facilities or local school. While you might assume the places where young children play or learn would be safe, many schools and childcare facilities have "significant and serious problems with indoor environmental contaminants," according to the Environmental Protection Agency.[67] Here's part of the problem: the majority of childcare providers have a poor understanding of potential sources of toxin exposure in their facilities and schools, according to recent research.[68] But I've found that voicing your concerns to administrators, managers, and owners about such chemical exposure at schools and childcare facilities can have an impact.

For example, when I noticed the use of conventional air fresheners, an intense smell of cleaning products, and no open windows at my son's daycare center, I emailed the CEO of the company (which owned more than two thousand daycare centers nationwide—a fact I didn't know at the time). Surprisingly, the CEO called me the next day and listened closely to my concerns. We set up a meeting with his team, after which they immediately started requiring daycare providers to undergo retraining on the proper use of cleaning chemicals and how to avoid dangerous mixture combinations.

When it comes to outdoor play spaces, avoid areas that specify they've been sprayed with pesticides, or call your town or city public works department to learn if your favorite playground is regularly sprayed with pesticides. Choose playgrounds that use cut grass and/or wood chips rather than padding made from rubber tires, because that padding has been made from petroleum-based products and, similar to artificial turf fields, contains many toxic chemicals. If your child is exposed to such material, wash their skin as soon as possible, using soap and water.

TEENAGERS

Puberty is the time when hormone activity is at its highest, as teens and preteens undergo incredible changes, like menstruation, body hair growth, breast development, sudden growth spurts, voice change, acne, and emotional and mood variability. Many of these changes are due to the surging levels of sex hormones like testosterone and estrogen. These sex hormones are highly susceptible to influence or alteration by EDCs—many EDCs, in fact, are estrogen mimickers, which means they imitate the hormone's actions in the body, increasing the risk of acne, early onset of puberty, thyroid dysfunction, cancer, diabetes, obesity, and development problems. For example, thyroid cancer has become the leading cause of pediatric endocrine cancers, accounting for more than 6 percent of all pediatric cancers from 2012 to 2016 and reflecting a recent rise in cases over the past four decades.[69]

Another way EDCs may be affecting teens is that young women all over the world are experiencing menarche (the onset of a menstrual cycle) at younger and younger ages than in previous decades.[70] What's more, teens develop new tissue in their reproductive and endocrine systems and their brains continue to grow until age twenty-five—and chemical exposure can interfere with how all these critical parts develop.

Teens also use more personal-care products like makeup, perfume or cologne, hair spray or gel, antiperspirant, scented moisturizers, shaving cream, and other items than do adults, increasing their exposure to single chemicals, as well as the potentially more noxious mixture of chemicals (as discussed in chapter 6).

What to do? The quality of personal-care products used by teens is critically important, so teach them how to buy with care. (You'll discover how to do this in chapter 6.) Studies show that using low-chemical cosmetics and other personal-care products for just three days can reduce the toxic chemical levels in a teen's urine by up to 45 percent![71] At the same time, encourage your teen to eat more organic food whenever possible and limit their consumption of canned drinks like soda and seltzer, which almost always contain the EDC bisphenol A (BPA) (see page 147 for more on this). These are the years when habits can form for life, so try to model and encourage nontoxic behaviors, like filtering your drinking water, avoiding chemical cleaners, and limiting your time on electronic devices. The latter can emit harmful low-level radiation, especially when placed near sensitive areas of the body like the groin, abdomen, and chest (see page 195 for more about this).

PRE-, PERI-, AND MENOPAUSAL WOMEN

The years before and during menopause are a critical time when it comes to exposure to environmental toxins, as this is when a woman's hormones go through drastic changes. Years of population research show that routine or everyday exposure to environmental chemicals, particularly EDCs, may cause an early onset of menopause, which has been linked to an increased risk of heart disease, depression, osteoporosis, and even premature death.[72] Toxin exposure during menopause may also intensify vasomotor symptoms of the condition, which is a fancy way of saying hot flashes and night sweats.[73]

What to do? Following the advice outlined in this book can significantly reduce your exposure to parabens, phthalates, PFAS, BPA, and other EDCs. While weight gain and the signs of aging can make some menopausal women want to reach for potentially toxic diet products or more cosmetics or other personal-care products marketed for aging (I can personally attest to this desire), don't get suckered into buying products that promise fast results for weight loss or say they're anti-aging; most of these claims are just marketing hype. One of the best ways to look and feel better is to lower your toxic exposure and improve your overall health.

HOW ENVIRONMENTAL TOXINS CAN IMPACT MULTIPLE GENERATIONS

The effects of environmental toxins on pregnant women are alarming enough. But what's downright shocking is how exposure to chemicals during pregnancy can affect not only an unborn child but also their children—and generations of children to come. While in the womb, a female fetus will develop her entire set of eggs and a male fetus will grow testes and sperm stem cells that create sperm during his lifetime. When women are exposed to environmental chemicals during pregnancy, it can alter those developing eggs or sperm stem cells in the unborn child, impacting the child's future offspring.[74] This is known as a *multigeneration effect*, which occurs when exposure during pregnancy affects the pregnant woman, her children, and her grandchildren.

Unfortunately, the insidiousness of environmental chemicals may extend beyond three generations, in a phenomenon known as *transgenerational effects*, which occur when generations beyond the direct exposure—a pregnant woman, her children, and her grandchildren—are impacted. Research on pregnant women shows that exposure to environmental chemicals during pregnancy can increase the disease risk in generations of offspring to come, affecting great-grandchildren, great-great grandchildren, and so on.[75] That's because toxic industrial chemicals have been shown to cause *epigenetic changes*, which mean they're capable of altering the way in which our genes work and express themselves. These alterations are then passed along to future generations. Toxins like vinclozolin, for example, an industrial chemical used to kill fungus, has been shown in animal studies to cause health effects in the offspring and grand-offspring of the mice originally exposed.

Another example is a medication called diethylstilbestrol (DES), which was prescribed to pregnant women in the United States between the 1930s and the 1970s to prevent miscarriage and pre-term delivery. Although the mothers themselves remained relatively unharmed by the medication, their daughters (known as "DES daughters") who were exposed in utero developed a variety of gynecologic health conditions, including reproductive organ malformations, infertility, breast cancer, and a rare kind of vaginal cancer.[76]

Before we move on to chapter 3, I want to share what happened with Ashley and Taylor, as their stories illustrate how small reductions in our daily exposure can make a big difference to our symptoms and overall health outlook.

For Ashley, who suffered from rheumatoid arthritis (RA) most likely spurred on by gut dysbiosis, I prescribed a six-day course of steroids to help quiet her painful symptoms. After the swelling had gone down in her hands and feet, we began to work on removing some "hits" to her microbiome. She started by opting for less processed forms of protein than the veggie burgers and plant protein powders she had been consuming almost daily, choosing instead foods like hard-boiled eggs, organic poultry, hummus, and quinoa. For the days she wanted to supplement with protein powder, she traded her old daily protein powder for a brand screened for contaminants and replaced her canned seltzer with filtered water flavored with a splash of organic juice that she drank out of glass or stainless-steel containers (and without a straw!). She also started filtering her water (which I talk more about in chapter 4).

I also suggested she begin to take a high-quality probiotic with the appropriate amount of colony-forming units (CFUs; as described in chapter 8) to help repopulate her gut with good microbes. In addition, I recommended she take a high-quality omega-3 fatty acid supplement with highly concentrated levels of EPA (eicosapentaenoic acid) and DHA (docosahexaenoic acid), which have been shown to reduce inflammation and joint pain in RA patients.[77] (Note the use of "high-quality": many supplements don't contain enough of the active ingredient in the serving size advertised, which is why finding high-quality, pharmaceutical-grade brands is key, as discussed beginning on page 227.)

We also discussed the use of over-the-counter pain medications like ibuprofen (Advil) and naproxen (Aleve), which can irritate the stomach and disrupt the gut microbiome, especially when taken often and without food to protect the stomach lining. I suggested she try to wean herself off these medications as she began to feel better.

Finally, we talked about ways to lower her stress, since chronic stress can negatively impact gut microbiota and trigger an immune system response.[78] Part of stress reduction and supporting her microbiome also meant prioritizing her sleep quality. Yes, the actual quality of your sleep (sleeping through the night mostly uninterrupted in a quiet, cool room), and not just the quantity of your sleep (how many hours), can impact the health of your gut microbiota.

Several months later, when Ashley came back to see me, her hands appeared normal, her morning stiffness had subsided, and she had considerably more energy, despite taking no OTC pain meds or other drugs and making no other changes to her daily routine other than diet and supplements. She still had a ways to go—gut dysbiosis doesn't occur overnight, and neither does it heal quickly—but we were able to sufficiently address her symptoms and significantly reduce her chemical exposure, with the goal of helping to heal her gut microbiome.

AS FOR TAYLOR, I suggested he start by keeping a metal fork, knife, spoon, cup, and stainless-steel or glass bottle in his travel bag so he didn't have to use plastic cutlery and coffee cups or drink from plastic water bottles while in the air. I recommended he eat a sit-down meal at a restaurant in the airport so he wouldn't be tempted by to-go food or heat-and-serve meals on the plane. While restaurant food isn't perfect, there's usually a greater variety of healthy options that aren't heated or served in plastic, the latter of which leaches obesogens from the food packaging and mobilizes them into the body.[79] We also discussed healthy snacks he could take in his travel bag, like raw almonds, hard-boiled eggs, dried vegetable chips, bananas, apples, and celery with hummus or almond butter, all of which he could easily keep in a stainless-steel container. When he wasn't flying, Taylor also started to eat organic whenever possible, opting for organic frozen veggies, which are usually less expensive and more nutritious when flash frozen than organic fresh veggies that may lose nutrients when shipped for long durations.

Four months later, when I saw Taylor again, he had already lost twenty pounds and was on his way to losing twenty more. While he made modest improvements to what or how much he ate, he had also become fastidious about which types of containers or wraps in which his food was served, in addition to the overall quality of his food choices. In other words, he focused on the chemical *quality* of his food and drinks, not just on the quantity or composition of calories, carbs, fat, and protein, which he was able to implement by taking small steps.

BOTH ASHLEY'S AND Taylor's stories show that taking simple steps to lower your exposure to common chemicals in your diet can have a big impact on a wide range of symptoms.

Chapter 2 Takeaways

- Your gut microbiome is the largest immune system organ in your body, and feeding it cleaner food and water, and reducing your overall environmental exposure, will help your healthy microbes thrive. Start today by picking up foods known to boost gut health but that don't include synthetic chemicals. Think organic or grass-fed yogurt (preferably sold in a glass container), organic raw sauerkraut, and organic garlic and onions, all of which contain healthy gut bacteria like probiotics and prebiotics.
- Common chemicals known as obesogens—found in food, water, food packaging, personal-care products, and home goods—can cause weight gain or prevent weight loss. Learning to become conscientious about chemicals can help energize your metabolism and speed weight loss. Start today by swapping any canned drinks (think seltzer) or food like canned beans for homemade items (carbonate your own seltzer or cook dried beans) or products sold in glass.
- If you suffer from headaches or migraines, try eliminating a common chemical to which you're regularly exposed to see if the occurrence subsides. Many people stop putting on synthetic perfume, drinking diet soda, or using conventional cleaning supplies only to discover their headaches go away.
- Are you pregnant? Are you the parent of a toddler, young child, or teen? Are you in or entering menopause? If you answered yes to any of these questions, it pays to be extra-vigilant about chemicals (using the tips given in this book), since exposure during these times can

be more detrimental. Start today by swapping out one conventional personal-care product like shampoo or body lotion, many of which contain endocrine-disrupting chemicals (EDCs) and immune-disrupting chemicals (IDCs), for a less toxic product per the EWG's Skin Deep Cosmetics database.

CHAPTER 3

How and Why Dangerous Environmental Chemicals Exist

HERE'S A SHOCKING fact that surprises everyone with whom I share it: more than ninety-five thousand chemicals are "approved" for commercial use in the United States today. Let that sink in for a second. That's nearly one hundred thousand chemicals in products many of us come into contact with every day.

The word *approved* might lead you to assume that a government agency or other regulatory body has tested these chemicals and made sure they are safe before they are allowed to come to market. But the vast majority of chemicals we ingest, absorb, breathe, or otherwise come into contact with on a daily basis have never been tested for safety, nor are they required to be tested by manufacturers before they are added to those products.

How did this happen? Let's take a look at the story behind how and why so many dangerous chemicals have ended up in our water, food, personal-care products, homes, and overall environment.

How Federal Agencies Overlook or Allow Toxins in Everyday Products

There are two federal agencies responsible for regulating the chemicals in our food and water: the Environmental Protection Agency (EPA) and the Food and Drug Administration (FDA). The EPA's job is to protect Americans from toxins in our air, soil, and water, while the FDA oversees the chemicals used in food, food packaging, bottled water, medications and medical devices, cosmetics, and some personal-care products. For consumer goods like toys, household appliances, and cleaning products, the US Consumer Product Safety Commission is in charge of regulating hazardous substances.

The EPA was granted the authority to regulate chemicals in 1976, when the United States passed the Toxic Substances Control Act (TSCA), a law intended to protect Americans from the overwhelming number of synthetic chemicals coming to market in the second half of the twentieth century. But out of the gate, the law failed to provide much protection, grandfathering in more than sixty thousand chemicals that could continue to be used without undergoing any testing.[1] Today, many of these "old" chemicals are still in use, even though most haven't been reviewed or analyzed for safety in decades.

In 2016, the TSCA was amended to require the EPA to review all new chemicals for safety, in the hope they could be made safe for use and handling by the public, especially among the most vulnerable populations, such as pregnant women, children, people with compromised immune systems, and the elderly. But since then, watchdog organizations like the Environmental Working Group (EWG)[2] and even the US Government Accountability Office (GAO)[3] have reported that the EPA has approved chemicals without adequate safety testing, while also missing most of its deadlines for safety review. At bare minimum, the EPA only has to review its laboratory tests and animal studies to identify which toxins raise the risk for developmental issues during and after pregnancy; additionally, it has to analyze the immune system effects and cancer risks of these toxins. Other testing can identify those concentration levels—also known as *maximum contaminant level* (MCL)—at which new chemicals are considered safe for consumption in drinking water. Of the tens of thousands of chemicals in use today, the EPA has halted production of fewer than ten and has banned even fewer for safety reasons.[4] Compare that to the actions of the European Union, which has banned around two thousand toxins from commercial use.[5]

Other laws designed to protect Americans from synthetic chemicals have also been largely ineffective. The Food Additives Amendment of 1958, for example, requires the FDA to prove a substance is safe before it can be added to food. But like the TSCA, the Food Additives Amendment included a clause that allowed thousands of existing additives to be grandfathered in; hence no safety testing. These additives were presumed to be *generally recognized as safe* (GRAS) because they had already been in use for years[6]—an invalid presumption for many reasons, including the fact that health effects from environmental toxins can take years to manifest. It's taken more than twenty years, for example, for some 9/11 survivors and first responders to develop cancers after being exposed to chemicals while working at Ground Zero.[7] Like the EPA, the FDA has come under fire from watchdog groups for failing to protect Americans from harmful chemicals.[8]

What about our tap water? The EPA oversees the establishment and enforcement of standards for the levels and kinds of contaminants in public drinking water, in accordance with the Safe Drinking Water Act of 1974. But setting standards and enforcing them are two wildly different things, and the failure of the EPA to do the latter is evident in public-water contamination crises like those in Flint, Michigan; Brady, Texas; and Newark, New Jersey, among other incidents. And these are just the cases of water contamination that have made it into the media spotlight. There are thousands of violations occurring every year that don't get publicized or remediated, and that often go unpunished or take years to rectify.[9] The Centers for Disease Control and Prevention (CDC) regularly measures the public's chemical exposures to many toxins, including PFAS, BPA, phthalates, glyphosate, and disinfection by-products, by testing the bodily fluids of Americans who take part in these ongoing biomonitoring surveys. Yet even though the CDC has found existent chemical levels in most people's blood or urine, this governmental agency, with its trademarked mission of "saving lives, protecting people," has done little to save or protect Americans.

How did we get into this crazy situation, where corporations are allowed to expose us to harmful chemicals nearly every hour of every day? In the United States, most of us presume the chemicals we encounter are safe until proven otherwise. And proving these toxins to be, well, toxic is laborious and timely (as detailed beginning on page 74), even if existing research shows a strong correlation between a certain chemical and an adverse health effect. Particularly, the onus of proving synthetic chemicals to be safe is on the federal government, not on the companies producing and using these chemicals. And with more than two thousand new synthetic substances coming to market every year, keeping pace with this waterworks of toxins is nearly impossible.[10]

In contrast, the European Union (EU) has some of the most extensive and protective laws on the books for environmental toxins. The EU follows the precautionary principle, which states that protective action should be taken against any product, action, or policy with a suspected risk of harm to people or the environment, even if that risk can't yet be scientifically proven.[11] In the United States the opposite is true, and substances suspected of causing harm are allowed willy-nilly in our food, water, personal-care products, and other items until any health risk can be exhaustively and conclusively substantiated by research.

Complicating matters is the fact that even when safety regulations do exist and are enforced, it doesn't necessarily mean the products are safe. The legal limit set by the EPA for contaminants in public drinking water, for example, can be hundreds of times higher than what scientists say may be harmful to our health.[12] The EPA also hasn't updated its legal limits on some contaminants in tap water for more than fifty years, making those standards archaic, scientifically obsolete, and arguably dangerous.[13]

The federal regulatory processes for chemicals in the United States are also slow-moving. Under the amended TSCA, for example, the EPA can review a minimum of twenty chemicals at a time, and each has a seven-year deadline for that review, with another five years for the chemical industry to comply with any new safety regulations set.[14] Even when scientists have published incriminating evidence on a certain chemical for years—such as research dating back to the 1960s that ties PFAS "forever chemicals" to significant health problems[15]—it can take the EPA just as long to set new safety standards.

The same is true of lead. For more than sixty years, the allowable levels of lead in drinking water have been dropping, but now we know there is no safe level of lead exposure. That is, the EPA, despite its stated goal of reaching 0 micrograms of lead in drinking water, has only reduced the allowable or action level of lead to 15 micrograms per liter, or 15 parts per billion, as compared to 50 micrograms per liter, which was the allowable level in 1975. The government also passed groundbreaking legislation in April 2024 to regulate and enforce new standards for perfluoroalkyls (PFAS) in drinking water, even though scientists have known for years that these toxic chemicals can add up, producing a lot of potential harm.

Finally, even when the federal regulatory process does work, the extent of its efficacy is extremely limited. Chemical companies can play a role in obfuscating the research by altering a synthetic substance after it's been on the market for years, so studies of the compound have to be performed again. A good example of this is bisphenol A (BPA), which is a common endocrine- and immune-disrupting chemical. After well-publicized studies linked BPA to diabetes, cancer, and developmental problems in children, among other health concerns,[16] BPA was banned in 2012 from use in plastic sports and baby bottles manufactured in the United States. But even when these extreme measures were taken, BPA was still allowed in thousands of products, including canned foods, printer paper, belts, bags, personal-care products, and cookware. Even worse, manufacturers of products that use BPA have created bisphenol analogs, which are similar-acting compounds varied enough that they no longer fall within the regulations applied to BPA. Some of these new compounds even have similar-sounding acronyms (BPS for bisphenol S, for example, and a derivative known as BPSIP) to skirt the regulations. These replacement chemicals, often called "regrettable substitutions" by toxic-chemical researchers, carry similar if not greater health risks.[17]

The Difficulty in Definitively Linking Chemicals to Health Conditions

As of this writing, there are only a few widely accepted environmental substances proven to *directly* cause human disease: cigarette smoking with lung cancer[18] and ultraviolet radiation with skin cancer.[19] These were rigorously proven scientific conclusions made after decades of exhaustive research. Otherwise, environmental toxins are said to have what's known as an "association" with a disease, meaning that the research suggests a relationship, but scientists can't definitively say that one causes the other. Causality is difficult to prove in any type of research, because scientists must be able to demonstrate that an independent variable causes a dependent outcome. But proving the causality between environmental toxins and diseases is even more challenging, for a number of reasons.

First, chemicals are difficult to trace and isolate because they're everywhere—in our air, water, food, homes, personal-care products, electronics—and most of us are subjected to thousands of toxins every day. Second, even if scientists could trace and isolate an individual's toxic exposure, people have different habits and genetic makeups that also influence their disease risk. Could scientists say, for example, that PFAS, which are possible carcinogens found in most tap water and other products,[20] are what is responsible for the recent uptick in early-onset cancers in the United States? Or is it phthalates, which are also linked to cancer and found in many personal-care products? Or could it be tied to the country's rising rates of stress, obesity, or processed food consumption? Our lifestyles are so complex and multilayered that it would be impossible to isolate the risk factors associated with any of those individual exposure points. Third, compounding the problem is that many lifestyle diseases, like cancer and heart disease, can take years to develop, making it difficult for researchers to pinpoint a certain time or exposure as what "caused" a person to get sick.

So, how do we know which environment factors are toxic and which are not? While scientists could answer more questions about environmental toxins and human health by conducting direct research on people, it's illegal and unethical to knowingly subject any human to potentially harmful substances. Instead, researchers have to rely on observations made on mice or other animals or performed on human cells or tissues that have been extracted and isolated in laboratories.

Epidemiological studies based on large groups or specific populations can also show links between chemical exposure and disease risk, but conclusions are difficult to draw because the larger the group studied, the greater the number of confounding factors, like varying lifestyles, genetics, and degrees of exposure over a lifetime. *Occupational studies*, which look at people exposed to toxins in the workplace, can be useful, even if limited. From occupational studies on firefighters and farm workers, for example, we know that flame retardants[21] and agricultural pesticides[22] can increase the risk of cancer in people.

IN SHORT, YOU can't rely on companies or the government to protect your health. History has shown that regulations, if any, work at a snail's pace, and we can't wait for legislation to change or more studies to be conducted when the evidence exists and we have reasonable solutions to implement change. While this conclusion may be alarming at first, I choose to see it as empowering, and I hope that you do as well. It's up to you to take control of your health now and to lower your risk of adverse health outcomes due to environmental toxins. You have the power to change how many chemicals you ingest, consume, absorb, touch, and even breathe in. All you have to do is step into your power and take back your health.

Chapter 3 Takeaways

- Just because food, tap water, and other consumer products are regulated by the US government, that doesn't mean they're safe. What to do? Keep reading: chapters 4 through 7 explain how to assess whether your food, drinking water, personal-care products, and home goods are safe and how to find safer products.
- Just because researchers can't definitively say synthetic chemicals cause disease, that doesn't mean they don't or won't cause disease.
- You can't rely on the government or manufacturers to protect you from environmental toxins, or even for more studies to be conducted. The evidence exists, and only you have the power to lower your chemical exposure and reduce your risk of environmentally driven disease. And those changes can start now.
- Remember this: *When an activity raises threat of harm to human health or the environment, precautionary measures should be taken, even if some cause-and-effect relationships are not fully established scientifically.* That's called the precautionary principle, used since the 1980s in developing policies and international treaties concerning human and environmental health.[23] In other words, better safe than sorry, look before you leap, and an ounce of prevention is worth a pound of cure.

SECTION II

AVOID

CHAPTER 4

What's Really in Your Water

YOU WOULD KNOW *if your water was contaminated.* Right? That's what Sofia heard over and over again after she moved from Ecuador to New York City more than twenty years ago. While she had grown up mistrustful of Ecuadorian drinking water, she believed her New York neighbors when they told her that their tap water, which came straight from a public treatment plant rather than a private well (the difference is explained in just a moment), was safe and clean. After all, her water didn't smell or taste bad, and New York City has always been one of the wealthiest cities in the world, with a population today of more than eight million.[1] Plus, don't all New Yorkers swear that the city's bagels are the best in the world because of their incredible water?

Sofia explained this rationale to me several years ago when, at age forty-six, she came to my medical office about her mouth ulcers. The first time we met, she arrived with her husband, James. It had been his idea, not his wife's, to make an appointment to see me about her mouth ulcers, which she had suffered from for years. While no doctor had been able to figure out what was causing them, James wasn't ready to give up, even if Sofia had resigned herself to living with them.

As I do with all patients, I listened closely to Sofia as she described her symptoms, the other health conditions she had, the prescription drugs she took and had taken in the past, and which measures or tests other doctors had previously prescribed. I then did a full physical exam and asked yet more questions, including whether she had any other symptoms, even if they were low-grade or seemed unrelated to her ulcers. Was she constantly tired, for example? Or always bloated? (The mouth is the first part of the gastrointestinal tract, so the health of the first can affect the health of the latter.) I wanted to know where she lived and had lived, the foods she ate, and of course, how much and *what kind* of water she drank daily. That's when she told me that, while she had always filtered her water in Ecuador, after moving to New York City, she drank right from the tap.

After we finished the exam, I recommended that we test Sofia's urine for heavy metals—specifically, for arsenic, lead, cadmium, and mercury—which is an easy screening that can be extremely informative and is oftentimes covered by health insurance, even though it's rarely ordered by doctors. In particular, I was concerned about Sofia's arsenic levels after learning that she drank a lot of unfiltered water and that her diet consisted largely of rice, which can have high levels of the heavy metal, even in organic and brown rice. I also suggested that Sofia have a biopsy to make sure her mouth ulcers weren't cancerous, which, astonishingly, no other doctor had ordered.

Sofia's biopsy results came back negative for cancer, thankfully, but as I suspected, her screening showed high levels of arsenic. Her results were 25 micrograms per liter (μg/L); for context, anything above 10 μg/L is considered toxic.[2] That meant the heavy metal could be the sole cause of her mouth ulcers. Fortunately, just because arsenic is ubiquitous, that doesn't mean it's complicated or costly to avoid, as I explained to Sofia. Resolving her mouth ulcers could be as easy as making a few dietary tweaks, the most important being to start filtering her drinking water the *right* way.

I emphasize the word "right" because, while a variety of filtering systems are capable of removing some or many contaminants from drinking water, some are more effective and aggressive than others, with the technology designed to remove hundreds of chemicals out of the thousands that can make their way into wells and public water systems.

Two months later, when we retested Sofia's arsenic levels, they had dropped to 17 μg/L; four months later, they were 13 μg/L, and her mouth ulcers had become less painful and occurring less frequently. After six months, her mouth ulcers were gone and her arsenic levels had dropped below 10 μg/L. This result was after no medications, no procedures, no other interventions—just filtering her water in a way that gets rid of arsenic and other toxins, while also reducing her rice consumption and cooking it only in filtered water (more on why and how this works beginning on page 86).

YOU MAY NOT be suffering from mouth ulcers as Sofia had, or have any other acute or chronic symptom or condition. But if you do, you may not think your drinking water could possibly have anything to do with it. Yet drinking contaminated water can cause both acute and chronic illnesses, including everything from hair loss, skin irritations, gastrointestinal issues, high cholesterol, and headaches to heart disease, pulmonary problems, neurological conditions, infertility, and birth defects and developmental problems in children—all of which research has linked to common toxins in drinking water.[3]

Of all the actionable advice in this book, learning what's in your water and how to filter it in the right way are the most critical steps you can take to protect yourself and your family. Drinking water is the *most* egregious, overlooked, undervalued source of human body contamination. In this chapter, you'll learn the most effective ways to make your drinking water safe—ways that are realistic, implementable, and relatively inexpensive. So, without further ado, let's get started.

Why Clean Water Matters

Some of the most common myths about drinking water include the following:

- Bottled water is healthier than tap water. FALSE.
- If you filter your water, you don't have to worry about contaminants. FALSE.
- Water from an office, home, or school watercooler is safe to drink. FALSE.
- If your tap water doesn't smell or taste bad, it's safe to drink. FALSE.
- The government regulates municipal water systems (from public systems rather than private wells), so you don't need to worry about the water. FALSE.
- The FDA regulates bottled water, so you don't need to worry about that. FALSE.

FAST FACTS ABOUT AMERICAN DRINKING WATER

- Tap water that contains chemicals that harm human health, including highly toxic PFAS, has been found in all fifty states.[4]
- Environmental toxins are found in many brands of bottled water, which may contain additional harmful compounds when bottled in plastic.[5]
- Despite the deficient regulation of contaminants in the US public water systems, there is no federal regulation requiring water filters or filtration systems that could remove microplastics and certain chemicals or even standards for filters to be effective.[6]
- Carbon water filters, like those found in popular water filtration pitchers and some refrigerator and on-faucet filters, don't remove many chemicals and may reduce others, like PFAS, by only 50 percent.[7]
- When water sits too long in some filtration systems, or the filter isn't changed in a timely or recommended fashion, chemicals can collect and contaminate the water to a greater degree.[8]

The safety and purity of our drinking water is one of the most relevant topics in human health and disease. By some estimates, up to 80 percent of all diseases and 50 percent of child deaths worldwide are related to poor water quality—it's why researchers say "the impact of water pollution on human health is significant."[9] While tap and bottled water in the United States and other Western countries is generally safer than that found in developing and underdeveloped nations, many of which lack sufficient water-treatment and sanitation infrastructures, American and European water is still rife with pollutants that can cause illness and disease.

It's important to understand why contaminated water is such a threat to human health; when you understand the "why," you'll be more likely to do the "what." So, let's get started.

Water is the largest substance by volume that we ingest and absorb. On a daily basis, Americans consume an average of up to four hundred gallons of water per household,[10] running the tap to drink, cook, bathe, brush our teeth, and wash our food, dishes, and clothes. We also absorb water from the foods we eat, even from those you wouldn't expect, like steak, chicken, and potatoes, all of which can contain more than 50 percent water. Nearly all fresh fruits and vegetables, like lettuce, spinach, zucchini, mushrooms, carrots, onions, watermelon, apples, and berries, contain more than 80 percent water. And if you cook them in water along with other absorbent foods like pasta, rice, or quinoa, that can increase their water content even more.[11]

Water is also the substance we consume with the greatest frequency. Each of us is like a walking, talking, breathing human sponge, sucking up and absorbing water (and everything in that water) every day, day after day, week after week, month after month, year after year, for the entirety of our lifetime. While some people may be able to go for weeks without food, nearly no one can survive more than several days without water. And because water is critical to the brain, making up 80 percent of the organ,[12] we also require water for all cognitive functions, like thinking, focusing, creating, coming up with new ideas, and even feeling joy and happiness, in addition to other human emotions.

The fact that our basic health and vitality are so dependent on water, however, has become a true crisis, given that the world's water today is "drowning in chemicals, waste, plastic, and other pollutants," according to the National Resources Defense Council (NRDC), an international, US-based environmental advocacy group.[13] To quote Christopher Weis, former senior toxicology advisor for the National Institute of Environmental Health Sciences, "increased vigilance for water security is needed to avoid catastrophic health occurrences."[14]

How Our Water Got Contaminated

While the earth is largely covered in water, 97 percent of it is saltwater, which scientists haven't learned how to convert into clean drinking water in a way that's easy, economical, and environmentally friendly.[15] Of the earth's remaining 3 percent freshwater, less than 1 percent can be used by humans and other living creatures. The rest is bound up in glaciers, ice caps, the atmosphere, and our soil, or has already been so polluted that it's incapable of being cleaned.[16] What this means is that there is very little precious potable freshwater on earth.

Roughly 80 percent of the United States's public drinking water comes from surface sources, like lakes, rivers, and streams. The remaining 20 percent comes from groundwater aquifers that supply wells, cisterns, and springs. In the US, industrial farming and other agricultural practices have contaminated both our groundwater and our surface water sources.[17] This contamination happens when toxins in insecticides, herbicides, fertilizers, and animal waste are absorbed by the ground, carried by rain or snowmelt into bodies of waters, or evaporated into the air, mixing with clouds or vapor only to fall back to the earth as precipitation. Industrial farming can also cause nutrient pollution, which occurs when too much nitrogen and phosphorus, found in chemical fertilizers and animal manure, sparks large growths of algae that can contaminate the drinking water. Nutrient pollution in groundwater at even low levels can be dangerous to people, making the issue "one of America's most widespread, costly, and challenging environmental problems," according to the EPA.[18]

Wastewater, which includes used water from household sinks, showers, and toilets (i.e., sewage), also pollutes our groundwater and lakes, rivers, and streams. In your own house or apartment, think of all the household cleaners, detergents, bleaches, and other chemical applications you may use to clean your sink, shower, and toilet, along with the dishes in your dishwasher and the laundry in your washing machine. These toxins all go down the drain, in addition to the chemicals in our cosmetics, skin lotions, shampoos, soaps, perfumes, and sunscreens that we wash off our skin. Add these chemicals to the pesticides on produce we may wash in sinks and, more notably, a host of prescription and over-the-counter drugs that we as human beings can't fully metabolize, including antibiotics, oral contraceptives, and antidepressants, causing us to excrete these chemicals in our urine and feces. For the vast majority of those homes that do not rely on septic tanks for waste removal, wastewater goes through treatment facilities before being released back into local waterways. But treatment systems can't filter out all the chemicals and toxins—which is why and how many end up in our groundwater and surface water sources.

Even more noxious than wastewater from homes, offices, and schools is the industrial wastewater produced by oil refineries, power plants, metal finishing facilities, food processing plants, fracking operations, and other industrial and commercial facilities, all which use noxious chemicals in high concentrations. The radioactive waste generated by mining, nuclear power plants, nuclear medicine, and the manufacturing and testing of military weapons, among other activities, also produces highly toxic wastewater. Adding insult to injury is that industrial wastewater, when mixed with chemicals from other wastewater sources, can create a chemical cocktail in our groundwater and lakes, rivers, and streams that may be even more dangerous than the impact of the individual chemicals we know of, according to research on this subject.[19]

The US sources for drinking water are also contaminated by stormwater runoff, which happens when rainfall washes oil, grease, road salts, and other chemicals from driveways, roofs, and paved streets into our water supply. Fuel spills and leaks also contribute significantly to water pollution; just one gallon of gasoline, in fact, can contaminate up to one million gallons of water.[20] Bigger spills can be even more detrimental, like the 1989 *Exxon Valdez* oil spill in Prince William Sound, Alaska, which dumped approximately 11 million gallons of crude oil into the bay, killing wildlife and halting the fishing industry. Today, some marine birds and mammals are still affected, and some fisheries haven't reopened—which is why, all in all, it's considered to be one of the largest environmental disasters in history.[21] And because everything in our environment and ecosystem is connected, any type of pollution, including air pollution, will eventually make its way into our water.

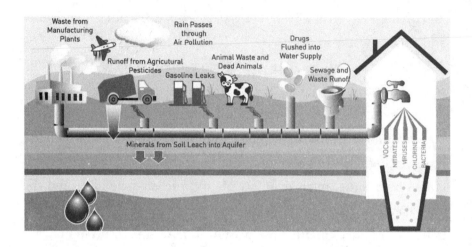

Constant contamination: How chemicals and other contaminants get into our drinking water.

Aly Cohen and Frederick vom Saal, *Non-Toxic: Guide to Living Healthy in a Chemical World* (Oxford, UK: Oxford University Press, 2020).

Before it comes out of your tap, contaminated water from lakes, streams, rivers, aquifers, and springs travels to a local wastewater treatment plant (there are 160,000 plants across the United States) to become tap water. Tap water is how approximately 80 percent of Americans get their drinking water (the other 20 percent gets their drinking water from underground wells).[22] Wastewater treatment plants use screens to remove large objects like twigs and garbage before sending the water through grit chambers that cause sand, grit, and other small particles to settle to the bottom. The water is then filtered through sedimentation tanks that remove smaller particles and is put through a system of secondary treatments that break down organic material. Finally, the water is treated with chlorine or other disinfectants to help kill bacteria.[23] While this process may sound rigorous, water treatment plants don't filter out many contaminants, including PFAS, microplastics, and plasticizers like bisphenol A (BPA); agricultural chemicals like glyphosate; and pharmaceutical drugs that wind up in the water; in addition to dozens of other chemicals.[24]

What's Really in the Tap Water?

By now, you're likely starting to see why our drinking water can be so contaminated—but what is it actually contaminated with? There are so many common chemicals in public drinking water—including lead, mercury, PFAS, chlorine, fluoride, pesticides, cleaning detergents, gasoline by-products, and pharmaceutical drugs—that it's impossible to list them all. What I can tell you with certainty is that many of these chemicals hamper the diversity and health of the microorganisms in our microbiome, affect the function of our brain cells, lower our immunity, shift our hormone activity, slow or alter the development in growing children, impair our insulin levels, and cause weight gain, among other effects. Some "forever chemicals" like PFAS, which are found in the majority of samples of US tap water,[25] don't break down over time—neither in the environment nor in our body. These chemicals make it difficult, if not impossible, for our body to detoxify and to maintain homeostasis, the body's preferred state of internal stability and function.

Despite the number of serious health effects and conditions caused by these environmental chemicals in our drinking water, few doctors recommend that patients consider or alter water consumption, much like they might do regarding their patients' diet, sleep, or exercise habits. While some doctors may instruct their patients to cut down on booze, sodium, or foods that contain bad cholesterol, or to take certain supplements, get more sleep, or start exercising, nearly no one in clinical medicine discusses what steps to take to mitigate one of the most significant and correctable factors of disease risk: our drinking water.

Because the United States enjoys a relatively extensive and modern sanitation and water treatment infrastructure, our tap water isn't as contaminated as it could be. We're also lucky enough not to have to drink rainwater, as people in other parts of the world do—especially since a team of Swedish researchers recently declared that all the rainwater on earth was unsafe to drink, owing to contamination with PFAS.[26]

Despite these advantages, the tap water from water treatment plants in the United States and many other developed countries is still contaminated with hundreds of chemicals, many times at unsafe levels. Here's why: drinking water that comes from public systems (as opposed to private wells) in the US is regulated by the EPA, a government organization that was given the authority to test and set the safety standards for tap water. As mentioned earlier, this legislation was the Safe Drinking Water Act of 1974; but that federal regulation of water has been woefully inadequate. There are three primary reasons for this:

The EPA doesn't have safety standards for most toxins. Of the ninety-five thousand human-made chemicals currently in commercial use, the EPA regulates only ninety or so found in tap water.[27] That doesn't mean that hundreds of other chemicals don't exist in drinking water—they do[28]—but the agency responsible for protecting the public's health doesn't have any safety standards for them. In fact, every year, more than two thousand new chemicals also enter the US market, yet despite this fact, the EPA hasn't set any new standards for toxins since 1996, other than finalizing limits on six "forever chemicals" in the PFAS group (out of the more than fifteen thousand known PFAS toxins[29]) in April 2024. Those new regulations will lower the allowable amount of PFAS, which are found in the tap water of all fifty states,[30] to much safer levels by 2029. But even in low doses, those PFAS have been linked to cancer, reproductive harm, immune system damage, and other serious health problems. And it will likely be years before new standards are set, whether for additional PFAS compounds or other kinds of chemicals.

The EPA's safety standards are insufficient. Of the ninety-plus contaminants the EPA does regulate, its safety standards aren't nearly strict enough, according to numerous scientists and public health agencies. First, the EPA's *maximum contaminant level* (MCL)—the highest amount of the contaminant legally allowed in drinking water—is based on a two-hundred-pound man who consumes two liters (about three quarts) of water daily. That makes these MCLs almost irrelevant for children and those who weigh significantly less. Many MCLs also haven't been updated in more than fifty years, despite overwhelming research suggesting that the permissible limit isn't safe.[31] All in all, many MCLs are hundreds of times higher than what today's scientists and public health agencies recommend as a maximum allowable level.[32] What's more, over the last several decades, the MCLs for many contaminants, like lead, have steadily been lowered based on accumulating research regarding adverse health effects.[33] What this means is that the levels of a chemical once designated as safe by the EPA *can* become regarded as unsafe, a development that corroborates why it's so important to filter water.

Safety standards for drinking water aren't always enforced. Despite their regulatory inadequacy, the EPA's standards for water do help make public drinking water safer—when those regulations are enforced. When they're not, though, we end up with contamination crises. Such crises haven't just occurred in Flint, Michigan; for example, between 2018 and 2020, 28 million people across the United States got their water from systems that, collectively, had been cited for 13 million violations of lead content, according to the NDRC.[34] Earlier reports by the same nonprofit show that 77 million Americans got their tap water from public water systems that had violated federal standards.[35]

National Primary Drinking Water Regulations

	Contaminant	MCL or TT (mg/L)	Potential health effects from long-term exposure above the MCL	Common sources of contaminant in drinking water	Public Health Goal (mg/L)
OC	Acrylamide	TT	Nervous system or blood problems; increased risk of cancer	Added to water during sewage/wastewater treatment	zero
OC	Alachlor	0.002	Eye, liver, kidney or spleen problems; anemia; increased risk of cancer	Runoff from herbicide used on row crops	zero
R	Alpha/photon emitters	15 picocuries per liter (pCi/L)	Increased risk of cancer	Erosion of natural deposits of certain minerals that are radioactive and may emit a form of radiation known as alpha radiation	zero
IOC	Antimony	0.006	Increase in blood cholesterol; decrease in blood sugar	Discharge from petroleum refineries; fire retardants; ceramics; electronics; solder	0.006
IOC	Arsenic	0.010	Skin damage or problems with circulatory systems; may have increased risk of cancer	Erosion of natural deposits; runoff from orchards; runoff from glass and electronics production wastes	zero
IOC	Asbestos (fibers >10 micrometers)	7 million fibers per liter (MFL)	Increased risk of developing benign intestinal polyps	Decay of asbestos cement in water mains; erosion of natural deposits	7 MFL
OC	Atrazine	0.003	Cardiovascular system or reproductive problems	Runoff from herbicide used on row crops	0.003
IOC	Barium	2	Increase in blood pressure	Discharge of drilling wastes; discharge from metal refineries; erosion of natural deposits	2
OC	Benzene	0.005	Anemia; decrease in blood platelets; increased risk of cancer	Discharge from factories; leaching from gas storage tanks and landfills	zero
OC	Benzo(a)pyrene (PAHs)	0.0002	Reproductive difficulties; increased risk of cancer	Leaching from linings of water storage tanks and distribution lines	zero
IOC	Beryllium	0.004	Intestinal lesions	Discharge from metal refineries and coal-burning factories, discharge from electrical, aerospace, and defense industries	0.004
R	Beta photon emitters	4 millirems per year	Increased risk of cancer	Decay of natural and man-made deposits of certain minerals that are radioactive and may emit forms of radiation known as photons and beta radiation	zero
DBP	Bromate	0.010	Increased risk of cancer	By-product of drinking water disinfection	zero
IOC	Cadmium	0.005	Kidney damage	Corrosion of galvanized pipes; erosion of natural deposits; discharge from metal refineries; runoff from waste batteries and paints	0.005
OC	Carbofuran	0.04	Problems with blood, nervous system, or reproductive system	Leaching of soil fumigant used on rice and alfalfa	0.04
OC	Carbon tetrachloride	0.005	Liver problems; increased risk of cancer	Discharge from chemical plants and other industrial activities	zero
D	Chloramines (as Cl)	MRDL=4.0	Eye/nose irritation; stomach discomfort; anemia	Water additive used to control microbes	MRDLG=4

OC	Chlordane	0.002	Liver or nervous system problems; increased risk of cancer	Residue of banned termiticide	zero
D	Chlorine (as Cl)	MRDL=4.0	Eye/nose irritation; stomach discomfort	Water additive used to control microbes	MRDLG=4
D	Chlorine dioxide (as ClO₂)	MRDL=0.8	Anemia; infants, young children, and fetuses of pregnant women: nervous system effects	Water additive used to control microbes	MRDLG=0.8
DBP	Chlorite	1.0	Anemia; infants, young children, and fetuses of pregnant women: nervous system effects	Byproduct of drinking water disinfection	0.8
OC	Chlorobenzene	0.1	Liver or kidney problems	Discharge from chemical and agricultural chemical factories	0.1
IOC	Chromium (total)	0.1	Allergic dermatitis	Discharge from steel and pulp mills; erosion of natural deposits	0.1
IOC	Copper	TT; Action Level=1.3	Short-term exposure: Gastrointestinal distress. Long-term exposure: Liver or kidney damage. People with Wilson's disease should consult their personal doctor if the amount of copper in their water exceeds the action level	Corrosion of household plumbing systems; erosion of natural deposits	1.3
M	*Cryptosporidium*	TT	Short-term exposure: Gastrointestinal illness (e.g., diarrhea, vomiting, cramps)	Human and animal fecal waste	zero

LEGEND

- **D** Disinfectant
- **IOC** Inorganic chemical
- **OC** Organic chemical
- **DBP** Disinfection by-product
- **M** Microorganism
- **R** Radionuclides

Limited list of primary drinking water contaminants and their maximum contaminant levels (MCLs). (For full list, go to http://nepis.epa.gov/Exe/ZyPURL.cgi?Dockey=P1005EJT.txt.)

It's obvious that the EPA doesn't adequately regulate the delivery of tap water in any meaningful way, which means the onus is on us to make sure our drinking water is safe.

PIPE DREAMS: THE SAFEST PLUMBING FOR YOUR HOME

Aside from treatment facilities, another factor that impacts the purity of public drinking water is the material and age of the pipes used to transport that water from those treatment facilities to our household faucets. There are more than 200 million miles of water pipes in the United States,[36] some which are old and made of lead, which is a toxic heavy metal that can leach from the pipe into the water flowing through it. Newer pipes are often made from polyvinyl chloride (PVC), a low-cost plastic that is a known carcinogen[37]—and those may be even more harmful than lead, according to reports.[38]

You can't do much about the public water pipes that bring the water to your home, but if you're a homeowner, you can replace any pipes within your house that were made with lead or PVC. The gold standard for safety, according to the Environmental Working Group, is copper piping, especially when it's paired with lead-free joint material.[39] Polypropylene is also a good choice, especially if cost is an issue; copper, while long lasting, can be pricey. Avoid pipes made from chlorinated polyvinyl chloride (CPVC), a close cousin of PVC that can also leach dangerous toxins into your water; and PEX, a polyurethane plastic that may shed petroleum by-products into your water.[40] No matter which material you choose, make sure all the pipe fittings, faucets, and other plumbing fixtures comply with lead-free national standards. If you're interested in replacing your pipes, find a licensed plumber who specializes in water-line work and can help you choose the best options for your situation. If you're buying a new home, ask the seller and realtor about the kind of water pipes in the house; while regulations vary from state to state, the seller should be required to disclose this information.

HOW TO FIND OUT WHAT'S IN YOUR WATER

The EPA requires most community water systems to provide their customers with an annual water quality report or consumer confidence report detailing the quality of the local drinking water for the past year. But many people who receive these reports often toss them aside as junk mail or find them too difficult to interpret, or even outdated (which they largely are).

To find out what's in your drinking water, visit the Environmental Working Group's Tap Water Database at https://www.ewg.org/tapwater/. You can plug in your zip code and get a comprehensive overview of what's in your water. The EWG's database obtains test results for both regulated and unregulated chemicals, making its index more inclusive than the EPA's overview. At the same time, the database is really just a snapshot of what's in your water; the EWG can't collect data on all possible contaminants in all local water systems, and the results can change on a daily basis owing to environmental factors.

However, the purpose of checking the database isn't to show you whether your water is safe or to what degree. Instead, it's to spur you to take action to filter your water once you see the kind of contaminants and chemicals known to be in your tap water. Even if you discover only a few contaminants in your area, dozens more may exist, meaning that your water can't be considered safe. Similarly, determining which contaminants are more harmful than others depends on a variety of factors. The end point is to understand that your tap water is, in fact, contaminated and that you should filter it.

Examples of the kind of chemicals commonly found in tap water include:

- Disinfectants and disinfection by-products
- Discarded pharmaceuticals
- Plasticizers, such as BPA and phthalates
- "Forever chemicals" like PFAS (found in nonstick pans, greaseproof paper, and waterproofing/stain guards)
- Antimicrobials, such as triclosan
- Industrial chemicals, such as benzene, toluene, vinyl chloride, carbon tetrachloride, and styrene (the main ingredient in Styrofoam)
- Coal ash and fracking chemicals
- Fragrance chemicals
- Agricultural chemicals, insecticides, fertilizers, and herbicides (e.g., cancer-causing glyphosate, the main ingredient in Roundup)
- Chemicals from discarded cosmetics, beauty products, and hair dyes
- PCBs (polychlorinated biphenyls, industrial chemicals found in the ocean and many other waterways)
- Plastic microfibers and microplastics
- Nanoparticles used in sunscreens, anti-odor fabrics, and as a method to treat drinking water for viruses

ALL ABOUT MICROPLASTICS

Microplastics may be super tiny, but these minuscule fragments are a massive deal when it comes to the water we drink—and to our health and world environment in general. Microplastics are produced when large plastic debris breaks down over time into smaller pieces, eventually ending up less than 5 millimeters in diameter—about the size of a sesame seed.[41] Microplastics are found not only in bottled water but also in tap water (although to a lesser degree than bottled water) and almost all other beverages and food.[42] And we don't just eat and drink microplastics; we also breathe them in our air, causing buildup in the lungs and consequent respiratory problems[43]—that's how ubiquitous they are in our environment. In fact, researchers have found microplastics on nearly every part of the earth, including in all our oceans, atop our isolated mountains, on remote beaches, and even in fresh Antarctic snow.[44] They have also been detected in more than 1,300 aquatic and terrestrial species of living creatures. For these reasons, microplastics have been found in 80 percent of the human blood tested,[45] as well as in our lungs, liver, kidneys, breast milk, feces, the fatty tissue of the neck vessels,[46] tissues of the penis,[47] testicles,[48] and maternal and fetal placental tissue.[49] Studies show that microplastics are now found in the brains of deceased humans, and concentrations are rising over time.[50]

This is hardly happy news, as microplastics have been shown to interfere with the body's microbiome, hormone levels, and cognitive function, in addition to ratcheting up inflammation, as immune cells attack the foreign particles when they enter our body.[51] What's more, avoiding microplastics is impossible—they're everywhere. But it's also why filtering the microplastics out of your drinking water is critical; it's one of the few proactive ways you can limit your exposure. While the efficacy of filters to remove microplastics is still debatable, the science of water filtration technology is also improving rapidly.

Thankfully, too, the government has begun to take action to limit microplastics. In 2015, President Obama signed into law the Microbead-Free Waters Act, which bans microbeads, a form of microplastics added to personal-care products to give them a scrubbing property and enhance their ability to exfoliate skin. Also, in 2022, California legislators approved the world's first requirements to test and report microplastics in sources of drinking water, paving the way for other states or countries to—we hope—follow suit.[52]

Water from Private Wells

As mentioned earlier, tap water supplied by public water systems is regulated by the EPA. But water from private wells—which is how approximately 20 percent of Americans get their tap water—isn't regulated by any federal agency.[53] Our federal government also doesn't require that private wells be tested for toxic chemicals unless an adjoining property is sold, at which point only limited chemical testing is mandated. This is especially troubling, since many private wells contain an overwhelming number of contaminants, including radioactive substances and heavy metals, according to the US Geological Survey.[54] No matter the results of a test of your well water, you should still filter your water the right way (as detailed beginning on page 107). If money is an issue, skip the annual testing and invest instead in an aggressive and effective filtration system for your home.

The quality of your well water can change significantly through the year, as it can be affected by dynamic factors like the agricultural/farming seasons, weather (e.g., flooding), and wavering water tables. The Centers for Disease Control and Prevention recommends you conduct annual maintenance and testing in the spring, when most areas of the country experience the highest rainfall (and therefore have the biggest potential for contamination).[55]

For an unbiased and independent analysis of your well water, order a testing kit provided by the laboratory network Tap Score, rather than a local water company, the latter of which may corner you into hooking up to their water system. Tap Score offers several different well-water tests that range from several hundred dollars to up to nearly $1,000 per test. Depending on how much money you want to spend, you can have just the essentials tested (heavy metals, minerals, hardness, bacteria) up to testing for a number of industrial and agricultural contaminants, including plasticizers and pesticides.

Otherwise, the EPA recommends calling your county health

department for well-water testing options—some counties may test well water for free—or finding a state-verified testing laboratory; the EPA provides a list of state-verified testing labs on its website.[56] The cost of annual maintenance and contaminant testing varies, but it can be expensive and is not necessarily covered by homeowners' insurance.

Fluoride and Chlorine: Toxins Intentionally Added to Public Tap Water

So far, we've talked only about unintentional contaminants that end up in our drinking water. But some chemicals, like fluoride and chlorine, are intentionally added by the government to our water, even though they have known health effects. For the last seventy-five years, the government has enriched tap water with fluoride after finding that children who drank fluoridated water had fewer cavities and less tooth decay.[57] In the United States today, approximately 75 percent of all tap water is fluoridated.[58] If you get your water from a private well, it likely also contains fluoride, because it is an element found in underground rock layers and groundwater.[59]

Recent research, however, shows that the fluoride in tap water poses bigger health risks than the gains from preventing a couple of cavities. It has been found to interfere with thyroid function,[60] trigger brain developmental issues,[61] and even lower IQ in school-age children.[62] Fluoride in drinking water has also been fingered for increasing the risk of dementia.[63] These are some of the reasons why many countries don't fluoridate their water, including Austria, Canada, Denmark, France, Germany, Greece, Mexico, and Switzerland, among other nations.[64]

The government also adds chlorine to our drinking water to help kill bacteria, viruses, and other microorganisms. But chlorine is noxious in high amounts, and has been shown to cause cancer and reproductive problems.[65] The chlorine can also mix with organic matter in the water to create disinfection by-products, which may be even more toxic than the chlorine itself.[66]

The solution to the presence of these chemicals in your tap water isn't to start drinking bottled water, which can also contain fluoride and chlorine. Instead, look into filtering your water in a way that removes both chemicals (as described on page 109).

What's Really in Bottled Water

Spoiler alert: The water found in individual bottles of water, as well as in the bottled stuff you can get out of a water cooler in your home or at the office, is oftentimes no less contaminated than the stuff that comes out of your tap, according to multiple sources.[67] In fact, bottled water can be even more contaminated than tap water, owing to higher concentrations of tiny plastic fragments known as microplastics (see page 99). In one study, microplastics were found in 93 percent of all bottled-water brands tested, including Aquafina, Nestle Pure Life, San Pellegrino, Dasani, and Evian.[68] Most single-use plastic bottles are also made from polyethylene (PET), which can leach eighty additional chemicals into the water.[69] What's more, lots of that bottled water comes from the same sources as our tap water—springs, wells, and surface sources. Many times, too, bottled water is just tap water pumped into a plastic container and sold on store shelves.[70]

If you think the EPA does a poor job regulating public tap water, the Food and Drug Administration (FDA), which is responsible for monitoring bottled water products, may be doing an even worse job, with fewer restrictions and less frequent testing, according to the environmental watchdog group Green America.[71] For example, while the EPA tests public drinking water one hundred times a month for coliform bacteria (think *E. coli* and similar bacteria that can cause gastrointestinal illness), the FDA analyzes bottled water only four times a month, on average.[72]

Just like our public drinking water, bottled water can contain hundreds of contaminants, sometimes at toxic levels. Even brands manufactured by seemingly trustworthy companies have been shown to include high levels of toxins. For example, a recent *Consumer Reports* survey found arsenic at levels just below the federal limit (and three times the amount recommended by the nonprofit) in Starkey Spring Water, which is manufactured by Whole Foods Market.[73] The same survey found detectable amounts of harmful PFAS in most of the forty-seven brands of both noncarbonated and carbonated bottled water it tested.[74] Another study by the Environmental Working Group found thirty-eight different contaminants, including industrial chemicals, bacteria, and trace pharmaceutical drugs, in all ten brands of bottled water tested.[75] While consuming these contaminants in one bottle of water won't cause disease per se, the cumulative effect, just like with tap water, can be harmful to your health over time.

Some companies bottle spring water, which comes from underground aquifers that naturally rise to the surface.[76] While spring water may sound clean, it can be highly toxic, with recent studies finding chemicals like arsenic and uranium in most untreated spring water.[77] Though manufacturers usually treat the spring water before bottling it, these treatments, similar to those conducted at public water facilities, don't remove all the chemicals and contaminants.

Bottled water has additional drawbacks that tap water doesn't have, including the fact that it's not cheap. According to the Environmental Working Group, bottled water costs two thousand times more than tap water, even though, in some instances, it's the exact same thing.[78] It's also not good for the earth, with researchers estimating that bottled water is 3,500 times worse for our environment than tap water, as both fossil fuels and precious clean water are needed to produce the plastic bottles, many of which can't be recycled.[79] In 2021 alone, used plastic water bottles helped contribute to 25 million tons of plastic waste.[80]

The bottom line is that bottled water, no matter which brand you buy or how much testing or purification processes the company boasts, is not good for you, for your wallet, or for the environment. The solution is not to wait for a brand that can bottle without contaminants but, rather, to filter your water the right way.

WHAT TO KNOW ABOUT ARSENIC IN WATER-RICH FOODS

Many foods, including seafood, mushrooms, and poultry, contain organic arsenic, although the highest concentrations are found in rice and products made from rice, like some cereals.[81] This type of naturally occurring arsenic is known as *organic arsenic* and is not nearly as toxic as *inorganic arsenic*, which is a by-product of industrial manufacturing and is also found in pesticides, animal feed, and some pharmaceuticals.[82] In the United States, the primary way we're exposed to dangerous inorganic arsenic is through contaminated drinking water.[83] In fact, arsenic has been detected above public-health guidelines in the drinking water in all fifty states, according to the Environmental Working Group. Making matters worse, many popular forms of water filtration, including Brita filters (the inexpensive plastic pitchers that many people keep in their fridge), aren't certified to remove the arsenic from tap water.[84] Bottled water isn't safe, either, as the heavy metal has been detected in many bottled brands, including those manufactured by Whole Foods, according to *Consumer Reports*.[85]

What You Need to Know About Filtering Your Water

If you're already using a water filter at home, pat yourself on the back: you've taken one of the most essential and actionable steps you can to reduce your exposure to environmental toxins. Filtering the water for drinking and cooking can significantly reduce your exposure to contaminants known to cause deleterious health effects. Regardless of whether you have your tap or well water regularly tested, or what your water supplier says about the content of your drinking water, you still need to filter your water, as taste and smell are no indicator of purity, home tests can't analyze all possible contaminants, and water-supplier reports are flimsy at best.

But not all water filters are created equal. They vary hugely by technology, cost, size, and type, as well as the degree of contaminants removed. They come in a multitude of varieties, like water pitchers, built-in refrigerator filters, faucet-mounted filters, countertop filters, under-sink filters, and even whole-home filtration systems, the latter of which are installed where the water main enters your home so that all the water that comes out of your taps, showerheads, and water-based appliances (think dishwashers and laundry machines) is filtered.

These choices are mind-muddling at best. To help you cut through the confusion, here's a quick primer on four common filtration technologies:

Activated carbon filters: Activated carbon, found in water pitchers, faucet-mounted models, and other filtration systems, works by chemically attracting and physically absorbing contaminants. There are two different types: carbon blocks and granulated activated carbon. Carbon blocks have a dense porous structure that filters water as it flows, while granulated activated carbon uses fine grains of activated carbon to remove contaminants. According to the Environmental Working Group, carbon blocks are typically more effective because they offer more surface area, but they are also more expensive and need to be replaced more regularly than granulated activated carbon.[86]

Contaminants removed: Activated carbon filters differ widely in the type of contaminants they target. Some filter out only chlorine and chlorinated by-products while others also reduce pesticides, lead, mercury, and volatile organic compounds (VOCs). Activated carbon filters, found in water pitchers, faucet filters, and filters built into refrigerator doors, generally don't remove bacteria, arsenic, fluoride, nitrates, and some other toxins, but they may eliminate up to 73 percent of PFAS, according to a study by scientists at Duke University and North Carolina State University, who note that the results vary significantly by filter brand, some of which had no effect on the "forever chemicals."[87] While there's no way to know for sure which contaminants and to what level an activated carbon filter removes them, whether you already own one or are considering buying one, you can read the claims made by the manufacturer. Just be sure to look for those that are third-party-tested and/or certified by the National Sanitation Foundation (NSF) or the Water Quality Association (WQA).

Ion exchange: This technology uses electrically charged molecules to remove the calcium and magnesium, which, when dissolved in drinking water in high quantities, are what make water "hard." Ion exchange is typically the technology used in water softeners, which are systems installed on faucets or at the head of a water main to counteract hard water. Some water softeners use sodium to help remove minerals, which can be problematic for those on a low-salt diet.

Contaminants removed: Ion exchange and water softeners remove minerals; some also take out barium and radium. However, water softeners won't remove bacteria, chlorine, PFAS, lead, arsenic, and most other chemicals.[88]

Distillers: Technically, distillers aren't filters. Instead, they remove contaminants by heating water to a high temperature, causing it to vaporize before condensing back into liquid, leaving behind some toxins. Distillers are less common than other types of home filtration systems.

Contaminants removed: Distillers generally remove bacteria and viruses, along with arsenic, lead, nitrate, and a handful of other contaminants. But distillers won't remove chlorine, VOCs, and many other toxins.[89]

Reverse osmosis (RO): Systems that use this technology reverse the flow of water through a semipermeable membrane that traps contaminants. Some reverse osmosis systems also include activated carbon filters. The RO membranes have an extremely small pore size, allowing them to filter single-cell organisms like bacteria and viruses, and particles as small as 1 micron (or 0.001 mm). They can be installed under your sink or as part of a whole-home system.

Contaminants removed: RO systems remove bacteria, viruses, and most chemical contaminants, including chlorine, arsenic, lead, fluoride, pharmaceuticals, and radioactive particles. According to the Duke University study, under-sink RO filters are also the most efficient way to remove PFAS, reducing the levels of these chemicals by as much as 94 percent.[90]

THERE ARE OTHER types of filtration technology, including ultraviolet treatment and ozone filters, but we won't cover them here because they're used primarily in whole-home systems, which I don't necessarily recommend. These systems can waste water, are expensive, and don't remove the same degree of contaminants as some of the technologies just discussed.

Choosing and Maintaining Your Water Filter System

Because reverse osmosis uses the most aggressive filtration technology available and removes the greatest number of contaminants, this technology is the gold standard for home use. In fact, RO technology is so superior that all dialysis machines must use regulated RO filtered water for patients, according to federal standards.[91] I know this because my father has been a practicing kidney specialist for more than sixty years and remembers when this stipulation was first mandated in the 1970s. I recommend to all my patients, regardless of their water quality or health concerns, that they install an under-sink RO system and use RO filtered water for drinking and cooking. *If you take only one actionable step to reduce your toxin exposure, install an RO filter*, as it's the easiest and most effective way to limit environmental chemicals in the substance we consume the most throughout life other than air.

Cost: On average, under-sink RO filters range from $200 to $1,000, which may not include the cost of installation. In general, more expensive filters will remove more contaminants and often carry extra certifications, but I remind readers that installing any filter is better than going without one, if cost is an issue. While RO filters are more expensive than a water pitcher, under-sink RO filters can last for a decade, mitigating the cost in comparison to replacing water pitchers with far more frequent filter replacements. Keep in mind that you'll have to replace the filter in any RO system per the manufacturer's recommendation or it won't be effective. The timeline to replace filters varies widely by which type of system you get—anywhere from six months to five years.

RO systems are also far less expensive over time than buying bottled water for your home, which as you now know is usually just as contaminated as tap water, if not more so. What's more, if you end up with a health condition from drinking contaminated water (like Sofia did), you may spend far more money on doctor copays and drugs. An under-sink RO system is a small investment to make for overall health and happiness. And in my opinion, good health is priceless. If you rent your place, you can still install an under-sink or countertop RO system, which a plumber can install within an hour and which can be taken out as quickly when you move out.

Other considerations: Every once in a while, a patient will say that they don't want to use an RO filter because it produces "dead water," meaning it contains no minerals. While RO filters do remove all nutrients, water is not a good source of nutrition, including minerals like calcium and magnesium, as they are better obtained and absorbed through food choices. Another concern I hear from patients is that RO filters use and discard large amounts of water while filtering and they can increase water bills. While older filters can, newer models are smaller and more efficient, and some recent models waste no water at all. When possible, opt for newer, more efficient models to limit water waste.

Beware of fakes: Buy RO filters and other systems only from authorized vendors to avoid counterfeit water filters, which are a real thing. In 2015, US Customs and Border Patrol seized more than five thousand fake refrigerator filters from China.[92] These fake water filters don't work and can even contain contaminants like arsenic. The National Sanitation Foundation warns consumers to look for incorrect labeling or packaging and to weigh the filters before purchasing, as counterfeit filters often weigh less than authentic ones.[93] Some brands allow you to search for authorized vendors by zip code on their website. You can also reduce the risk of buying counterfeit filters by looking for National Sanitation Foundation and Water Quality Association certifications on a product.[94] Finally, if the price is too good to be true, it probably is.

Maintain your filtration system: An RO filtration system is only as effective as the semipermeable membrane that comes with it. Many big-box stores outsource membrane manufacturing to other countries while still carrying a "Made in America" label. To avoid this trap, look for an RO system rated by *Consumer Reports* and also certified by the National Sanitation Foundation. These qualifications are critical no matter which filtration system you choose, including water pitchers, countertop filters, or showerhead filters.

Change the filter in your system as often as the manufacturer recommends. Otherwise, your water will be just as contaminated, if not more so, than unfiltered tap water. Old filters will stop working and can also become breeding grounds for bacteria.[95] Also, store any pitchers and detachable filters in the refrigerator when not in use to reduce the potential for microorganisms to grow in the filter.

SHOULD YOU FILTER YOUR SHOWER WATER?

While filtering your water for drinking and cooking is a priority, I also recommend installing mounted filters on showerheads, which you can add to most standard showerheads and should cost only around $25 each. They are worth the investment, not only for your physical health but also for that of your skin and hair. Every time you shower, you inhale chlorine and other chemicals as the water vaporizes, which affects health. Chlorine and heavy metals in the water can also strip natural oils from skin and hair.[96] Opt for showerhead filters certified by the NSF that also work well at high temperatures.

HOW GOOD ARE BUILT-IN REFRIGERATOR FILTERS?

Drinking and cooking with water filtered by a built-in refrigerator system is safer than using water straight from the tap, as long as you change the filter per manufacturer recommendations. That's because refrigerator filters often use activated carbon, which helps remove PFAS and other chemicals.[97] But no refrigerator filter will remove as many contaminants as an RO system. If you prefer the convenience of a refrigerator filter and/or like using the ice machine but want your ice to be created from filtered water, you can purchase inexpensive tubing that a plumber can then connect to a reverse-osmosis filtration system. Contact your appliance company for more information and next steps.

Extra Tips for Safer, Cleaner Water

The following are some smart ways to improve the quality of your tap water. Just remember that these tips shouldn't take the place of filter installation.

- Let the water run at full flow from the tap for ten seconds to flush out pollutants like lead and bacteria that can attach to or grow on faucet components. Then, reduce your faucet to half-flow before filling your glass or container for cooking. If you don't want to waste water or you live in a drought-stricken region like California, capture the extra water and use it on nonedible plants.
- Hot water from the tap contains more contaminants than cold water, as toxins like lead detach more easily from plumbing surfaces when they're exposed to high temperatures. Instead, fill a teapot or cauldron with cold water and heat the water on the stove.
- Avoid drinking water from five-gallon blue carboy water containers, like those found in office watercoolers. They are usually made from polycarbonate, which releases BPA into the water. You can check for this yourself by using the recycling code chart on page 146. If you see the number 7 inside a triangle anywhere on the container, it likely is made from BPA or a toxic replacement.
- When traveling by plane, don't drink the airline's coffee, tea, or water or accept drinks with ice unless you are sure all the water comes from a sealed bottle (this is one of the instances when bottled water is a better choice). The airline industry isn't required to regularly test the water in its tanks. A 2019 study found that water served on many major and regional US carriers was significantly unhealthy, prompting researchers to advise travelers to "never drink any water onboard that isn't in a sealed bottle" and to even avoid washing your hands in the bathroom, opting instead for hand sanitizer.[98]

As discussed in this chapter, paying attention to your water quality by filtering what you drink and what you use for cooking is one of the easiest and most effective ways to lower your chemical exposure and protect your health and well-being. You wouldn't inhale fumes from an exhaust pipe, bathe in gasoline, or eat foods known to contain industrial chemicals, pharmaceuticals, harmful bacteria, and radioactive particles, would you? Yet so many of us drink and consume poisonous water all day, every day. You don't have to let that contaminated water interfere with your health; the solution is simple, and the power is in your hands.

Chapter 4 Takeaways

- Stop drinking tap water, well water, and bottled drinking water, all which can contain an unknown number and concentration of toxins. Opt instead for filtered water.
- Invest in a reverse-osmosis water system for your kitchen sink or even entire home plumbing. If price is an issue, investing in any filtration system is a worthwhile move that can help significantly lower your environmental exposure.
- Filter your drinking water at home and take it in a stainless-steel canister to the office and out to restaurants, two places that oftentimes don't filter drinking water (remember that bottled water is oftentimes just as toxic).
- Filter the water you cook with, since industrial contaminants in tap water will end up in your food.
- Consider installing a filter for your shower: Your skin is your body's biggest organ, and it can absorb a lot during a warm, pore-opening shower. Using showerheads with a carbon block filter, in addition to an RO kitchen filter, can effectively reduce your toxin exposure without breaking the bank.
- Consider replacing your home's water pipes with a cleaner alternative if they are old or made from plastic.
- Rethink your drinking water, as it is one of the most effective actions you can take to do your body good!

CHAPTER 5

What's Really in Your Food

MELISSA THOUGHT SHE should feel as though she were on top of the world. Having graduated two years ago as an all-star student athlete from her university, the twenty-four-year-old had just landed her first real job as an architectural associate at a prestigious firm. Life was exciting, and she was ready to embrace it. So, why on earth did she feel as though she could barely get out of bed? And how had she managed to gain twenty pounds in the last six months, despite continuing to work out regularly?

These questions prompted Melissa to make an appointment to see me, as she grew more and more concerned that there was something seriously wrong with her. She was also worried about her hair. "Is it normal to lose *this* much?" she asked, showing me the hairbrush she had brought into my medical office as evidence. She also wanted to know why her knees and hips were so stiff, even though she had stopped training competitively after college.

Unfortunately, Melissa's symptoms weren't unusual. In recent years, I've seen more and more patients at increasingly younger ages with the same aggregate of low energy, weight gain, hair loss, and generalized joint pain. While this combo can indicate a number of conditions, in Melissa's case—as is true for millions of Americans—the problem was *hypothyroidism*, also known as having an underactive thyroid, which occurs when the body's thyroid gland doesn't make enough thyroid hormone to support normal function. Patients with hypothyroidism may also experience irregular menstrual cycles, be intolerant of the cold, have dry skin, and suffer periods of depression.

In the last decade, the incidence of hypothyroidism and other thyroid conditions, like Hashimoto's disease, has increased significantly in the United States, even among those like Melissa who don't have a family history of thyroid problems.[1] If you're not familiar with Hashimoto's, it's an autoimmune condition that triggers the immune system to attack the thyroid gland, manifesting in many of the same symptoms as rheumatoid arthritis and lupus, and oftentimes progresses to hypothyroidism. While the level of incidence of Hashimoto's is unknown, five out of every one hundred Americans develop hypothyroidism.[2] As a rheumatologist, I spend a lot of time diagnosing and treating autoimmune conditions like Hashimoto's, many occurrences of which are aggravated or caused by *immune-disrupting chemicals* (IDCs). But I also see a lot of thyroid cases that aren't autoimmune, which can also be aggravated or caused by IDCs or *endocrine-disrupting chemicals* (EDCs). More often than not, though, environmental toxins are *both* IDCs and EDCs, sharing the ability to throw a body into a turmoil of dysfunction and decline.

When it comes to thyroid health, the thousands of IDCs and EDCs in what we drink and eat every day can pull a double whammy—interfering with our immune system and thyroid function while also sabotaging our levels of iodine, an essential trace mineral that the body needs to make the thyroid hormone.[3] There's more about iodine in chapter 8, but what to know now is that many of us don't get enough of this mineral, as our intake of iodine-fortified salt has declined in recent years, and many of us don't eat enough foods that are naturally high in the nutrient (like seaweed, seafood, eggs, and milk-based dairy products).[4] At the same time, our exposure to synthetic chemicals known to interfere with iodine uptake has only skyrocketed. It's essentially a double-edged sword. Not only are many of us nutritionally deficient in iodine, but we're also bombarded with IDCs that bond to thyroid gland cells, interfering with our iodine storage and transport, both which we need for optimal thyroid-hormone production.

Melissa, who didn't know she had hypothyroidism before seeing me, had spent years prioritizing lean protein, as do lots of athletes. More recently, she'd also started a low-carb diet to lose the weight she'd gained, increasing her intake of lean protein and vegetables as a result. While these choices are certainly healthy, conventional poultry and veggies are almost always washed in hypochlorite bleach, done to help reduce the spread of harmful bacteria like *E. coli*.[5] While that's a positive when it works (the jury is still out on the efficacy of food washes), hypochlorite bleach can also degrade into perchlorate, a toxic chemical shown to cause neurological problems and disrupt thyroid function by preventing iodine uptake.[6]

After starting her full-time job, Melissa had begun to eat more deli turkey and chicken meat, which she found was a more convenient way to get her protein than cooking or preparing it herself. But while convenient, processed meats—a list that also includes ham, sausage, and bacon—can contain added nitrates, which are synthetic chemicals known to increase the risk of cancer and also inhibit iodine uptake.[7] Nitrates only compound thyroid problems. Five years earlier, Melissa had also stopped using iodized table salt in favor of sea salt and Himalayan pink salt, and was therefore no longer consuming the mineral. And while store-bought bread is also often fortified with iodine, it wasn't part of Melissa's new low-carb diet.

Many traditional doctors would have prescribed Melissa thyroid medication to treat her hypothyroidism. But as an integrative medicine physician, I believe that lifestyle changes are more effective than prescription drugs for most non-life-threatening conditions, as medications oftentimes mask symptoms while failing to address the root cause of illness. What's more, many modern ailments can be triggered or aggravated by lifestyle habits, meaning that if a patient doesn't change their lifestyle, they won't fully or effectively treat their illness.

In Melissa's instance, she was already doing many things right. She was filtering her water, prioritizing sleep, exercising regularly, and using mostly clean products on her body and at home. And while her diet was healthy "on paper," she was unknowingly consuming a ton of synthetic chemicals that were harming her thyroid. Yet these could be reduced with just a few easy tweaks. For this reason, I recommended to Melissa that she:

- Prioritize consuming organic poultry and produce whenever affordable and accessible.
- Buy only "nitrate-free" deli meat while reducing her overall consumption of processed meats.
- Swap excessive animal protein (e.g., chicken and other meats) for wild-caught seafood and plant-based proteins like organic beans and nut butters when possible.
- Take a daily multivitamin with adequate amounts of iodine and selenium, along with the three other fundamental "fertilizer" supplements I recommend to combat environmental exposure (more on this beginning on page 226).
- Continue to exercise regularly, since it's one of the most effective ways to detox environmental chemicals (as explained in chapter 8).
- Continue to prioritize sleep, since it's one of the most effective ways to detox environmental chemicals (as discussed in chapter 8).

Melissa followed my advice, and when I saw her again three months later, her thyroid hormone levels had normalized, her energy levels had improved twofold according to her self-assessment, her hair loss had stabilized, and she'd lost seven pounds, despite making no other changes to her diet. After six months' time, she'd lost another three pounds and reported feeling like her "normal" self again, ready to engage in her new life. Better still, she had learned the playbook on how to reduce environmental toxins in her diet without giving up the foods she loves the most.

THIS IS NOT to say that reducing your exposure to dietary chemicals will solve every medical ailment. Treating health conditions is a complex matrix that often includes many different factors and solutions. But as you'll learn in this chapter, thousands of synthetic and toxic chemicals hide in the foods and drinks we consume every day, many of which are easy to avoid. If we do choose to continue to ingest them, however, these toxins can influence our health by directly affecting our gut microbiome—the trillions of microbes that live in our intestinal tract and direct nearly every physical function in our body and brain. Chemicals in our food supply, just like those in our water, can also erode the gut's delicate lining, causing inflammation and triggering leaky gut syndrome. (A reminder from chapter 2: This occurs when our intestinal barrier becomes so compromised that toxins cross the stomach's vulnerable epithelial lining and enter the bloodstream, where they travel straight to our cells, organs, and other tissue.)

While drinking clean water is a priority because you consume more water by volume than any other substance, reducing your dietary intake of toxins is the second-best way to reduce your overall toxic intake. And ideally, you do both: you filter your water *and* you make safer food choices. In this chapter, you'll discover the surprising truth about what's really in your food and you'll learn the easiest and most effective ways to avoid those harmful dietary toxins.

The Problem with Processed Foods: Toxic in More Ways than You May Think

Most of us eat and drink hundreds of chemicals every day. These chemicals reside in both processed foods and healthy whole ones like fresh produce, unprocessed meats, fresh dairy, wild-caught seafood, dried beans and legumes, unrefined grains, and raw nuts and seeds.

Even adopting a Mediterranean diet, which prioritizes fresh whole foods, won't save you from toxin exposure. But organic matters: a recent study found that those who followed a nonorganic, conventional Mediterranean diet—meaning the foods eaten were not organic—consumed up to four times the environmental contaminants as those who followed a northern European diet.[8] Still, there's a critical caveat: when those study participants switched to an all-organic Mediterranean diet, meaning they ate only organic foods, their chemical exposure dropped by 90 percent.[9]

Before we get into the toxins lurking in fresh whole foods, let's tackle the bigger elephant in the room: the chemicals found in processed foods. By volume, most Americans eat far more processed foods, which are foods that have been altered from their natural state in some way, than healthy whole ones. In fact, 60 percent of Americans' average caloric intake comes from ultra-processed food and drinks.[10] Those ultra-processed foods include those you'd expect, like fast-food burgers, store-bought chips, packaged cookies, frozen meals, soda, and other obvious offenders. But the term also encompasses many foods and drinks that we don't typically think of as refined: nondairy milks, flavored yogurts, packaged bread, protein bars, meat substitutes, store-bought smoothies and juices, granola and muesli, and countless other items. While most food is processed in some way—cooking rice and freezing fresh vegetables are considered forms of processing, for example—the most processed foods contain hundreds of chemicals. Many of those chemicals have been associated with a range of adverse health effects at "exceedingly low, chronic levels of exposure," according to authoritative research.[11] Adding insult to injury, processed food is almost always packaged in boxes, bags, tubs, tubes, wraps, wrappers, cartons, and other containers made from dangerous toxins that can and do leach into what we eat and drink.

The US Food and Drug Administration (FDA), an agency with the stated mission of protecting the public's health, allows more than ten thousand chemicals to exist in processed foods that are sold today.[12] These chemicals, more broadly known as food additives, include artificial preservatives, artificial flavorings, artificial colors, synthetic sweeteners, lab-made emulsifiers, engineered oils, and other synthetic substances designed to alter or enhance a food's flavor, texture, smell, color, mouthfeel, shelf life, or other attribute. About half of these ten thousand chemicals are indirect food additives—substances that end up in the food and drink owing to the processing equipment or after they leach out of the packaging.

While some food additives serve important purposes, many of them, whether added in the processing or leached from the packaging, are toxic to human health, especially when ingested on a regular basis over time. While these chemicals are allowed by the FDA, many have been linked to cancer, obesity, heart disease, growth and developmental problems, hormone ailments, reproductive issues, and cognitive disorders like ADHD.[13] And this describes only what we *know* about those food additives; many common chemicals found in what we eat and drink have *never* been tested for safety or have undergone only limited safety testing.[14] What's more, even if a food additive has been found to cause adverse health effects—like in the instance of perchlorate—the FDA has allowed it to remain in use.[15]

What gives? The laws applying to food additives in the United States are outdated and ineffective, to say the least. In 1958, Congress passed the Food Additives Amendment to the Food, Drugs, and Cosmetic Act of 1938, with the intention of protecting Americans from a burgeoning number of new chemicals. But since then, the law has provided more loopholes for food manufacturers than protection for Americans. The amendment, which was written to give the FDA authority to regulate food additives, grandfathers in hundreds of chemicals that were already in use, exempting them from testing.[16] Eighty-five years ago, when the law was first passed, there were only eight hundred food additives in use, not the ten-thousand-plus that exist today.[17] Most regrettably, the 1958 amendment included a disastrous provision that allows additives *generally recognized as safe* (GRAS) to be exempt from safety testing.

But the FDA doesn't decide if an additive is GRAS—a food manufacturer does.[18] This has allowed hundreds of chemicals to flood our food supply without undergoing any safety testing at all. In fact, nearly 99 percent of all new food chemicals produced since the year 2000 have been allowed to enter the food supply without any safety testing or FDA analysis.[19] What this means is that just because an additive is approved or allowed to be used in our food, it doesn't mean it's safe for human consumption. And independent testing of many GRAS ingredients has shown that they may cause disease and disability.[20]

In addition, a recent evaluation by independent researchers found no evidence that the GRAS panels, which determine the safety of GRAS-labeled ingredients, adhere to FDA guidance and oftentimes are rife with conflicts of interest, with members putting "the health of Americans at risk."[21]

What to do? While fresh, whole foods can harbor many chemical contaminants, as will be explored shortly, most contain few to no food additives, including the ten-thousand-plus chemicals mentioned so far. Whole foods also have a lower risk of contamination by toxins from processing equipment and packaging. And because whole foods typically spoil much more quickly, they don't usually sit for long on hot trucks, in warehouses, or on store shelves, reducing the likelihood of and degree to which any chemicals in the plastic, Styrofoam, or other packaging may leach into the products.

When you do eat processed food—as is inevitable for almost everyone, including me—you can lower your toxin exposure by opting for certified organic products whenever possible and affordable (see page 137 for tips on buying organic without breaking the bank). Per the US Department of Agriculture, certified organic products can't contain most synthetic food additives, including many artificial preservatives, colors, and flavors—USDA-certified inspectors actually visit farms and businesses to make sure products meet standards. Organic packaged foods also can't have genetically modified (GM) ingredients, lessening the risk they'll contain high levels of pesticides like glyphosate.

Glyphosate is the most widely used herbicide in the world, used pervasively in US agriculture and found in residential gardening products like Roundup. Glyphosate has been linked to cancer, among other ailments.[22] If you do eat conventional foods, it's important to know that glyphosate is detectable in almost all packaged goods made from soy, corn, and wheat, including pizza, pasta, crackers, and cereal, and more than 95 percent of all oat-based products.[23]

When organic isn't affordable or available, examine the product's ingredient label carefully, avoiding products with additives listed that you can't pronounce, especially those included in my discussion of the Most Toxic Immune-Disrupting Chemicals to Avoid in Processed Foods (beginning on page 130). Finally, choose packaged products, whether organic or conventional, that are sold in glass containers, which will reduce your exposure to food-contact chemicals (discussed further beginning on page 145).

THE TRUTH ABOUT GENETICALLY MODIFIED ORGANISMS (GMOS)

Genetically modified (GM) foods have been a hot topic of debate for decades. Some argue that artificially manipulating the genes of plants—which is what genetic modification does—is smart science, helping make crops more disease resistant, nutritious, and produce greater yields, which can help feed the world's burgeoning population.[24] But others, like me, point to the fact that GM crops, when engineered to be pesticide tolerant, require greater applications of toxic herbicides and insecticides (including glyphosate) while failing to produce greater yields, per independent studies.[25]

More worrisome, an overwhelming body of research suggests there may be adverse health effects from consuming GM foods, including an increased risk of asthma, allergies, and immune system dysfunction.[26] There's also concern that consuming products made with GM crops that have been altered to be antibiotic resistant could negatively impact our gut microbiome, increasing people's antibiotic resistance as well.[27]

At the same time, the effects of consuming GM foods aren't fully understood. Their impact on human health hasn't been studied long enough, with some researchers comparing GMOs to the insecticide DDT, which the government banned only after years of use and when conclusive evidence finally showed it causes cancer.[28]

Today, foods that contain GMOs must be labeled "bioengineered" or "derived from bioengineering," which is misleading language at best. Unfortunately, loopholes in the labeling law, which was passed by Congress in 2016 and went into full effect in 2022, still allow some products with

GM ingredients to forgo any designation.[29] The only way to completely avoid GMOs is to buy certified-organic products; by law, these can't contain GM ingredients. Or you can opt for items labeled "Non-GMO Project Verified."[30] Because 90 percent of all soy and corn in the United States has been genetically modified to be pesticide tolerant,[31] I especially discourage consumption of these crops and their ingredient by-products, like cornstarch and soybean oil, unless they're labeled non-GMO.

THE MOST TOXIC IMMUNE-DISRUPTING CHEMICALS TO AVOID IN PROCESSED FOODS

Of the thousands of possible chemical contaminants in food, for some there is more conclusive evidence suggesting they cause harm to human health. The following is a list of immune-disrupting (IDCs) and endocrine-disrupting chemicals (EDCs) that have been recognized by the Environmental Working Group (EWG) and/or the states of California and New York as particularly toxic for human consumption. If your favorite food or drink contains any of the following ingredients—all are required to be listed on food labels—swap it for an alternative that doesn't include it. For a list of healthy swaps, see Appendix 1, my list of one hundred foods to have in your shopping cart (page 287). And while the following list isn't exhaustive by any means, it's a great starting place to limit your toxin exposure whenever consuming conventionally processed products.

Artificial colors (synthetic food dyes): For years, synthetic food dyes have made media headlines for increasing the risk of cancer and behavioral problems like hyperactivity, among other ailments.[32] *Red No. 40, Yellow No. 5,* and *Yellow No. 6*, which account for 90 percent of all dyes used in foods and drinks today, contain benzidine, a known carcinogen.[33] Whenever these artificial colors are included in food or drinks in the European Union, the products must carry the warning label, "May have an adverse effect on activity and attention span in children."[34] *Red No. 3*, used in cake icing, chewing gum, and candy, is so potentially harmful that the states of California and New York want to ban it from all the products (the FDA banned Red No. 3 from use in cosmetics in 1990).[35]

Potassium bromate: Found in baked goods like bread, tortillas, and cookies, potassium bromate is a possible carcinogen that may also damage DNA and increase the risk of leaky gut syndrome (see chapter 2).[36] The chemical is banned in the United Kingdom, the European Union, Canada, and Brazil and must carry a warning label when used in food products sold in California.[37]

Brominated vegetable oil (BVO): Typically found in soda and juice, BVO has been linked to neurological conditions like the loss of muscle coordination and memory, in addition to thyroid problems.[38] BVO is already banned in Europe, while both California and New York are seeking to prohibit its use. While Coca-Cola and Pepsi Co. have stopped including the chemical in their families of products, it can still be found in smaller-brand items.[39] In July 2024, the FDA declared that BVO was no longer allowed in food, but the rule will not take effect for a full year, allowing companies to reformulate, relabel, and use up existing BVO-containing inventory before the FDA begins enforcing the regulation.

Artificial sweeteners: While noncaloric sweeteners like *acesulfame potassium, aspartame, erythritol,* and *sucralose* have long been favorites of dieters and others trying to stay trim, studies show that these artificial sweeteners can cause weight gain, in addition to diabetes, heart attack, stroke, and other metabolic issues, by interfering with hormone health and function.[40] Artificial sweeteners have also been shown to disrupt the delicate balance of bacteria in the gut microbiome and mess with insulin levels, ratcheting up hunger and glucose intolerance as a result.[41]

Titanium dioxide: Found in candy, baked goods, creamy salad dressing, and some frozen products like pizza and ice cream, titanium dioxide helps enhance color, whiten food, and prevent caking. But the chemical, banned by the European Union in 2022, can damage the immune system and our DNA—which is why California and New York are also looking to prohibit its use.[42]

Artificial preservatives: The FDA allows many different synthetic preservatives in food, some of which are more toxic than others. To help identify the most noxious, consider avoiding the following five, all of which are on the EWG's "Dirty Dozen" list of food additives:

Nitrates and nitrites, found in deli meats, hot dogs, and other processed meat and linked to cancer, thyroid problems, and other health issues.

Butylated hydroxyanisole (BHA), found in cured meats, breakfast cereals, potato chips, butter, beer, and other foods and identified as a possible carcinogen.

Butylated hydroxytoluene (BHT), found in breakfast cereals, chewing gum, baked goods, and other foods and identified as a possible carcinogen.

Tert-butylhydroquinone (TBHQ), found in crackers, microwave popcorn, and other snacks and linked to lower immune health and function.

Propylparaben, found in pastries, trail mix, tortillas, and other foods and linked to developmental and reproductive issues.[43]

Playing Pesticide Roulette: What to Know About Chemicals in Produce, Nuts, Grains, and Other Crops

There's no question about it: Unprocessed whole foods, like fresh fruit and vegetables, beans and legumes, nuts and seeds, and unrefined grains like oats and rice, are *much healthier* than processed foods. They contain fewer environmental toxins on average and boast far more hunger-satiating, health-sustaining, disease-fighting nutrients. By definition, *whole foods* undergo little to no processing and contain no food additives, which reduces exposure to thousands of possible chemical contaminants.[44] Unlike processed foods, whole foods also don't include added sugars, unhealthy fats, or synthetic carbohydrates. Prioritizing the consumption of whole produce and other plants, whether conventionally or organically grown, is essential for good health, with fresh fruits, veggies, beans, nuts, and whole grains providing natural and more bioavailable fiber, protein, fat, vitamins, minerals, and antioxidants than processed foods.[45]

That said, consuming a conventional version of the Mediterranean diet can expose you to a number of environmental chemicals—namely, pesticides, which are used liberally and oftentimes carelessly on conventional crops in the United States. American farmers are allowed to spray thousands of pesticides on their crops raised for food or animal feed, with virtually no testing for human or animal safety, nor any labeling attached that would let consumers know about that spraying. While eighty-five pesticides are prohibited for use in other countries for safety reasons, they are all used in the United States; in fact, these controversial chemicals account for one-fourth of the one-billion-plus pounds of herbicides, insecticides, and other pesticides used in the US every year.[46] Today, 90 percent of all Americans have detectable levels of pesticides or pesticide by-products in their urine or blood.[47]

That's a big problem, since many pesticides are known IDCs, meaning they can disrupt the function of the immune system, changing how critical immune cells work while stoking inflammation throughout the body.[48] This is one reason why pesticide residues in food have also been linked to allergies, asthma, and Parkinson's disease (which may have an autoimmunity component[49]), along with cancer, diabetes, heart disease, reproductive disorders, DNA damage, fertility issues, headaches, and other ailments.[50] People with the highest pesticide exposure are also three times more likely to die from cardiovascular disease than those with lower exposure, according to research, while children with the most pesticide exposure are more likely to be diagnosed with attention deficit hyperactivity disorder (ADHD).[51]

What to do? The most effective way to lower your exposure to harmful pesticides is to consume only USDA-certified organic produce, beans, grains, nuts, and other plants, which by law cannot be grown with synthetic chemicals. I may sound like a broken record, repeating the blessed sounds of organic food, but eating only organically grown food even for *just six days* can reduce the number of pesticide biomarkers in your urine by up to 60 percent, according to researchers at the University of California at Berkeley.[52]

When it comes to harmful pesticides, our greatest source of exposure is conventionally grown fruits and vegetables.[53] But that doesn't mean every fruit and vegetable you buy has to be organic. To make things easier, download the EWG's Dirty Dozen and Clean 15 guides to your smartphone; these guides are based on USDA analyses and are published annually to help consumers discern which fruits and veggies contain the largest and smallest pesticide residue levels on their surfaces, respectively. While the list changes slightly every year, at time of publication, the Dirty Dozen and Clean 15 lists include (in order of detectable pesticide residue or lack thereof) the following:

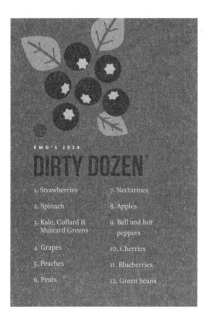
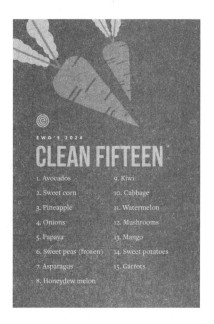

Source: Environmental Working Group, EWG.org

It's important to remember that herbs, while not included on the EWG's Dirty Dozen list, can also be contaminated with high levels of pesticides. For example, USDA testing has found that fresh cilantro can be contaminated with just as many pesticides as spinach or kale, the latter two of which are both top-three offenders on the Dirty Dozen list.[54] If you consume herbs frequently or in high quantities, opt for organic or grow your own.

You will also lower your toxin exposure significantly if you choose organic when buying other plant foods, regardless of whether they're on the Dirty Dozen list. These include beans, legumes, nuts, and whole grains like rice, wheat, and oats. All can contain pesticides, particularly glyphosate, that have shown to increase the risk of inflammation, developmental problems, and immune- and nervous-system dysfunction, among other ailments.[55]

WHY TO WASH YOUR PRODUCE AND HOW TO DO IT THE RIGHT WAY

Studies show that rinsing your produce with filtered water before you eat, prepare, or cook it can significantly reduce any pesticide residues.[56] To get the most bang for your buck, use a mixture of one teaspoon baking soda and two cups filtered water in a bowl. Add the produce and soak and agitate it for at least two and up to fifteen minutes, then rinse off with clean filtered water.[57] You can also mix one part white vinegar and four parts clean water to soak the produce for the same amount of time. Just never wash your produce with bleach, synthetic soap, or other harsh chemicals, which can end up being absorbed by those fruits and veggies and, ultimately, by you.

HOW TO EAT CLEAN IN A DIRTY WORLD WITHOUT BREAKING THE BANK

Opt for organic for the items you eat most frequently or in the greatest quantities. If you eat yogurt every day or often consume several servings of leafy greens at a time, choosing organic for these items is more important than getting an organic chicken or beef cut if you rarely eat meat. Eating organic doesn't just cut your chemical consumption; it can also increase your nutrient intake, as studies show that organic produce may contain more antioxidants, while organic meats, dairy, and eggs are often higher in omega-3 fatty acids.[58]

Start in the freezer aisle. Frozen organic fruits, vegetables, meats, and wild-caught fish are usually less expensive than their fresh counterparts and, in the instance of organic produce, they may contain greater nutrients because they are typically frozen immediately after being picked. When you buy frozen, you also don't have to worry about food going bad before you can use it.

Avoid the dirty dozen. When organic produce isn't accessible or affordable, stick to fruits and veggies listed on the EWG's Clean 15 (see page 135).

Buy in-season seafood and produce. In-season fruits and vegetables are fresher, often less expensive, and may contain greater nutrients than those flown in from parts of the world miles away. The same goes for seafood, since most varieties are caught or harvested according to a seasonal cycle. When you vary what you eat by the season (rather than consuming the same foods year-round), you also expose yourself to a wider variety of nutrients, which is better for your health. In-season foods are also more eco-friendly, leaving a smaller carbon footprint than foods shipped from great distances.

Bulk up. Buying organic nuts, seeds, beans, lentils, nut butters, coffee, and whole grains like oats, rice, and popcorn in bulk is usually cheaper than picking up packaged versions of the same items. Buying in bulk also lowers the risk of contamination from food packaging. Store the products in a glass or stainless-steel container instead of the plastic bags provided by stores.

Swap for what's on sale. I love a good grocery list just as much as anyone else does, but I've learned to make last-minute swaps if and when a different organic item is on sale when I'm shopping. For example, if I planned on picking up spinach for my salad but organic kale is available at a much better price, I'll always substitute.

Choose local. Buying local reduces the risk of food-contact chemicals that can leach into foods when those products sit for too long in plastic packaging in trucks and warehouses. Prioritizing local foods and drinks also supports your community and local economy.

Visit a farmers' market. Farmers' markets are a great way to buy both in-season *and* local foods and drinks.

HOW TO USE PLU CODES TO GET THE SAFEST PRODUCE

You know that little sticker with a bunch of numbers that you have to peel off apples, potatoes, and other produce? Well, you can use it to make smarter choices when you're shopping for fruits and veggies. Look for PLU codes that begin with the number 9, indicating they're USDA-certified organic, while avoiding produce with PLU codes that start with the numbers 3 or 4, which means they were conventionally grown. PLU codes that begin with the number 8 indicate genetically modified (GM) fruits and veggies, but this designation isn't mandatory, so any produce you pick up without an 8 code could still be GM unless it's USDA-certified organic.[59]

Clean Protein: What You Need to Know About Meat, Seafood, Dairy, and Eggs

Many patients ask me, "What's the most important item to eat organic? Is buying organic produce more important than organic red meat? Is organic cereal or organic chocolate really that essential?" My answer to them is the same as I say here: Whatever you eat the most frequently or in the greatest quantities is what you should prioritize buying organic.

That said, conventional meats, dairy, eggs, and seafood pose some real concerns. If you eat any of these animal or seafood products regularly—meaning at least once a week—here's what you need to know.

Cow's meat and diary: Conventionally raised cattle are often given growth hormones, steroids, and antibiotics. They're fed an unnatural diet of industrially produced grain feed that is often sprayed with pesticides like glyphosate and contains heavy metals such as arsenic, along with chemicals like PFAS and polychlorinated biphenyls (PCBs).[60] For all these reasons, trace amounts of pesticides, antibiotics, and hormones have been found in both cow's meat and dairy.[61] Conventional cow's meat and dairy, like other conventionally raised animal products, can also have higher traces of multidrug-resistant organisms than items from organically raised animals.[62]

Poultry meat and eggs: By law, conventionally raised poultry cannot be given hormones, but these chickens, turkeys, and ducks eat the same kind of industrially grown, chemical-rich feed that cattle do. Conventional poultry are also given antibiotics, and that's why researchers have found significantly higher levels of antibiotic-resistant bacteria in conventionally raised chicken than in organically raised animals. Most chickens are also kept in crowded, cramped conditions. Buying "cage-free" eggs is no guarantee that the birds were given anything more than a cramped indoor space to roam. Instead, research companies online and choose those that promote sustainable farming and/or transparent farming practices.

Pork: Similar to poultry, conventionally raised hogs cannot be fed hormones, but they consume the same industrial feed as do cows and chickens. What's more, conventionally raised pigs are often given ractopamine, a drug that helps animals put on muscle quickly but that experts say hasn't been adequately vetted for safety—which is why it's banned in the European Union and several other countries.[63] In US supermarkets, though, an estimated 80 percent of all pork products come from pigs that have been given ractopamine.[64] You can tell if pigs or cows have been given ractopamine by looking at the USDA website and searching for its official list of approved "Never Been Fed Beta Agonists" producers; this list names companies that don't feed animals this medication.[65]

Seafood: Fish and shellfish, no matter where or how they're caught or raised, can contain heavy metals like mercury, along with PCBs, dioxins, pesticides, PFAS, and other industrial chemicals.[66] That's because our oceans, rivers, lakes, and streams are that polluted. Unfortunately, what you or a friend might catch in a local lake isn't likely to be cleaner. Consuming just one serving of freshwater fish per year, such as a fillet of perch or freshwater bass, is equivalent to drinking water heavily polluted with PFAS chemicals for one full month, according to one study.[67] Emerging research also suggests that a lot of seafood can contain microplastics, those tiny pieces of plastic debris ubiquitous in our oceans, air, and all across the world that can cause harmful effects to human health.[68]

HOW TO BUY AND PREPARE SAFER MEAT, SEAFOOD, AND DAIRY

Hormones, steroids, antibiotics, ractopamine, mercury, microplastics, pesticides, PCBs, PFAS . . . the list of possible contaminants in animal meat and seafood is long and terrifying. Thankfully, there are evidence-backed, effective ways to reduce your intake of environmental chemicals in meat, seafood, and dairy. Here are my top four tips:

Buy organic animal meat, dairy, eggs, and other products made from animal meats, milk, or other ingredients whenever possible. When organic isn't accessible or available, choose grass-fed or pasture-raised products, which, while not as good as organic, contain fewer chemical contaminants than conventional products.

Before preparing meat or seafood, trim the fat, as fatty tissue is where many environmental toxins like PCBs accumulate and get stored.[69] For this reason, choose leaner cuts of meat and smaller types of fish. The acronym SMASH, which stands for sardines, mackerel, anchovies, salmon, and herring, can help you remember safe fish choices. In general, the fattier the meat or larger the fish, like swordfish, marlin, shark, king mackerel, and tilefish, the more chemicals it likely contains.[70]

When grilling meat, poultry, or seafood, marinate it in oil and spices, particularly dried or fresh rosemary, for at least thirty minutes to reduce the formation of cancer-causing compounds known as heterocyclic amines (HCAs).[71] Seasoning steaks, chicken breasts, chicken thighs, and fish fillets with black pepper also helps limit HCAs.

In general (but not always), farmed-raised seafood contains more chemical contaminants, as do larger, longer-living fish like sea bass and swordfish. When possible, choose wild-caught and smaller varieties from cold waters, such as salmon, mackerel, anchovies, sardines, and herring.[72] Other types of fish and shellfish can be safe choices, too, but it depends on where and how they're sourced. Unfortunately, buying "organic" seafood isn't any assurance, since the designation isn't official.[73] Instead, look for wild-caught or sustainably farm-raised seafood. To find out if a particular seafood is safe, go to the Environmental Defense Fund's Seafood Selector, at seafood.edf.org, and click to see which choices are both eco-friendly and healthy.[74]

WHAT FOOD LABELS REALLY MEAN

These days, just about every food product and drink, whether whole or processed, has stickers, labels, logos, or some other kind of "health" marketing term on its packaging. Here's a snapshot of what some popular labels actually mean:

USDA 100% organic: All ingredients are certified organic, including processing aids like cornstarch.

USDA organic: All ingredients, except those specified as allowable by the USDA, are certified organic. If you see this label on meat, dairy, or eggs, the animals must have been raised in conditions that allow for natural behaviors (room to graze, for example), have been fed 100 percent organic feed and forage, and have been given no antibiotics or hormones.[75]

Made with organic: At least 70 percent of this product contains organic ingredients.

Natural, all natural, or 100% natural: These designations aren't defined or regulated by the USDA or FDA, which means a food manufacturer can determine what's "natural," giving the description little value.[76]

Non-GMO project verified: This product contains less than 0.9 percent GMOs.[77]

Grass fed: This product comes from animals that were fed grass their entire lives, with no grain or grain by-products, and were also allowed continuous access to pasture.[78]

Grass finished: This product was produced from animals that were fed a mixture of grass and industrial grain.[79]

Cage-free: This designation for eggs means that the eggs are from hens that weren't technically kept in cages but could still have been raised indoors in crowded conditions.[80]

Free range: This product comes from animals that had continuous, free access to the outdoors for more than half their lives.[81]

Pasture raised: This product comes from animals that had continuous, free access to the outdoors for "a significant portion" of their lives.[82]

The Surprising Truth About Toxins in Food Packaging

The chemicals in our food may be frightening, but the toxins found in the synthetic packaging that surrounds and contains what we eat and drink are downright terrifying. To date, there are thousands upon thousands of known food-contact chemicals (FCCs), a broad term that describes toxins found in food packaging, food-processing equipment, and cook- and tableware, all of which can and do move into our food and drink. Of the more than twelve thousand FCCs known to exist worldwide, at least three thousand have been shown to be harmful to human health.[83] Many, though, have never been tested for safety. Of the FCCs that have been tested, like bisphenol A (BPA) and phthalates, many are both endocrine-disrupting chemicals (EDCs) and immune-disrupting chemicals (IDCs) that are capable of causing adverse health effects at "very low" levels for which "no safe thresholds are thought to exist," according to scientists.[84] The risks of exposure to FCCs include an increased likelihood of cancer, diabetes, obesity, neurological disorders like Alzheimer's, and autoimmune diseases.[85]

Researchers also warn that no one can predict the health effects when FCCs mix with other chemicals that are found in food and food packaging, creating potentially more dangerous chemical compounds in a phenomenon known as *mixture toxicity*.[86] What's more, since the US government doesn't require manufacturers to list the chemicals in their food packaging, most of us have no idea what we may actually be eating and drinking.

Although you can't easily identify the FCCs in food packaging, it's safe to assume that if a product's packaging isn't made from glass, stainless steel, or wax paper, it's loaded with FCCs. Beyond that, here are some other effective ways to reduce your exposure to these harmful toxins:

- Many food containers and cartons have recycling codes, also known as *plastic resin codes*, which are those tiny numbers inside triangles on bottles, bags, jugs, jars, tubs, trays, wraps, cups, and plates. While they weren't designed for this reason, the plastic resin codes can help consumers identify harmful food packaging. In short, avoid vinyl (#3), polystyrene (#6), and the dubious "other" (#7), the last of which usually contains BPA or just as harmful BPA substitutes like bisphenol S (BPS) or bisphenol F (BPF). To remember these numbers, tell yourself, "5, 4, 1, and 2; all the rest are bad for you." Note that 1, 2, 4, and 5 aren't chemical-free by any means—they are simply less toxic than the other choices.

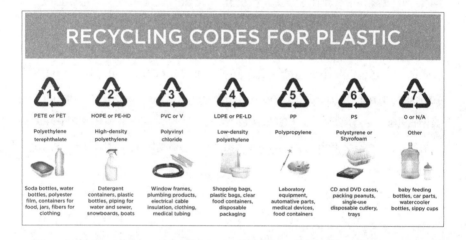

- Paper packaging, like takeout boxes, salad bowls, and sandwich wrappers, may appear to be more eco-friendly than plastic, but it contains high levels of PFAS, or "forever chemicals"; that's one reason why scientists have found higher PFAS levels in people who eat out often.[87] In 2024, the FDA announced that grease-proofing materials with PFAS can no longer be sold for use in food packaging in the US, but the phaseout is voluntary.[88] For this reason, avoid paper packaging whenever possible, which also includes pizza boxes, fast-food wrappers, microwave popcorn bags, and paper pet-food bags. If you eat takeout often, keep an extra set of glass or stainless-steel containers in your car or office, and ask restaurants to use those instead of their plastic, paper, or Styrofoam bowls or boxes. If you can't avoid fast-food wrappers or pizza boxes, remove the food as quickly as possible, especially if it's still hot.

- Most canned foods and drinks in the United States, including "healthy" soups, seltzers, vegetables, tuna fish, anchovies, and sardines, are in containers lined with BPA, which can migrate into the food. One study found that people who ate just one can of soup daily for lunch had a 1,000 percent increase in their urinary BPA levels.[89] While BPA-free cans may seem like the answer, many of those contain alternatives like BPS and BPF, which are just as harmful.[90] For this reason, limit your consumption of canned foods and drinks, including those that are organic, prioritizing fresh or frozen USDA-certified organic foods instead.

- If you've ever run Tupperware or other plastic containers through the dishwasher only to watch them get cloudy or opaque after a few washings, you're witnessing the degradation of plastic from high temperatures. Degraded plastic can leach chemicals into foods and liquids, especially acidic ones like tomatoes, citrus fruits, soft drinks, and certain dairy or high-fat items like meat, eggs, and oily foods.[91] For this reason, never put plastic containers in the dishwasher or microwave—even items that say they're dishwasher- or microwave-safe (this only means they won't melt at high heat).[92] Avoid microwaving any frozen vegetables that are sold in steamer bags, even organic vegetables. Instead, remove them from the bag and place them in a glass container, cover it with a paper towel if necessary, and microwave. Never consume drinks or food in plastic that has been exposed to heat like direct sunlight or in a hot car for prolonged periods of time.

- Styrofoam contains polystyrene, a suspected carcinogen that breaks down at high heat, leaching into coffee, tea, and takeout foods.[93] For this reason, avoid all Styrofoam and use glass containers or stainless-steel bottles for hot foods and liquids.
- Tea bags made from nylon or polyethylene terephthalate (PET) can leach billions of tiny plastic particles (microplastics).[94] Look for brands that aren't made from these materials, or invest in loose-leaf tea and brew it yourself with a stainless-steel strainer.
- Foods sold in bulk have fewer FCCs. Bring your own wax paper bags, glass, or stainless-steel containers to the store to avoid using their plastic bags. You can zero out the scale before weighing your purchases.
- Don't store food in glazed pottery, especially if that pottery originated from outside the United States, owing to possible lead contamination.[95]
- Many nonstick pans contain PFAS; those that claim to be free of PTFE and PFOA—two types of PFAS—can still include measurable amounts of toxic chemicals.[96] Skip the nonstick and opt for stainless steel or cast-iron pans.
- Antimicrobial cutting boards, cutlery, and other cookware may sound like a smart way to reduce bacterial contamination, but the synthetic antimicrobials like triclosan found in these products can be both EDCs and IDCs.[97]

Another Way We Ingest Toxins: Crazy Chemicals in Medicines

Today's pharmaceuticals are nothing short of marvels of modern science, saving millions of lives while increasing the quality of life for millions more. Some diseases, like chronic heart disease, kidney disease, some cancers, and HIV, among other ailments, that were once considered death sentences are now manageable conditions, all thanks to drugs. As a doctor, I've seen the evolution of drug therapies for patients with autoimmune or immune-suppression conditions that dramatically reduce the risk for death, debilitating pain, physical disability, and loss of income, while exponentially increasing the patients' quality of life. But there's another side to the story.

Many drugs, whether prescription or over-the-counter, are two-faced. They must affect the immune system to some degree in order to address a certain condition, but because they do this, they also often act as harmful immune-disrupting chemicals (IDCs) in the body, triggering trouble elsewhere. For example, the popular antibiotic minocycline, prescribed to treat Lyme disease, acne, and other skin conditions, is one of more than forty medications known to be IDCs, and they can cause immune issues (although mostly benign in nature) as a result. In the instance of minocycline, the drug can induce a condition known as drug-induced lupus, triggering joint pain, joint swelling, skin rash, hair loss, and fatigue.[98] Immunity tests performed on patients with these symptoms who take minocycline will show a problem with their immune system, prompting doctors to diagnose them with systemic lupus, when in fact the minocycline is the only reason for their symptoms and test results (and in most cases, when they stop taking the medication, their symptoms resolve without long-term implications).[99]

In addition to medications that can act as IDCs, many medications interfere with the gut microbiome, disturbing our delicate ecosystem of microbes by reducing good bacteria and stimulating the bad stuff to grow. A study of nearly 1,200 pharmaceuticals found that 24 percent of drugs blocked the growth of at least one important bacterial species in the gut.[100] In addition to antibiotics, examples of medications known to negatively affect the microbiome include those for blood pressure, acid reflux, diabetes, depression and anxiety, and pain—and specifically nonsteroid anti-inflammatory drugs (NSAIDs) like ibuprofen (Advil, Motrin, Midol, etc.). Taking ibuprofen may even kill as much good gut bacteria as a course of antibiotics, according to a study in the journal *Microbiome*.[101]

NSAIDs pose problems for the immune system, too. These painkillers, which include aspirin and acetaminophen (Tylenol), have been shown to lower immunity, which can increase susceptibility to infectious disease and make vaccines less effective.[102] Taking NSAIDs while pregnant can also boost the risk of birth defects and developmental problems.[103]

What's more, many pills boast plastic coatings made from phthalates, synthetic dyes, and preservatives, none of which you want to swallow on a daily basis if you can help it.[104] This is why I always advise patients to use prescription and over-the-counter medications only when essential. Talk to your doctor about why you may need medication, what the side effects are, and what your goals are. In general, it's best to use the fewest prescription and OTC medications at the lowest dose possible for the shortest time that you can. Discuss with your healthcare practitioner the goals and endpoints of your medication, possible natural substitutes, and a plan, if suitable, to get off the medications when appropriate.

AFTER THE KIND of water you drink, the foods you eat (and in what ways they're packaged) are primary sources of toxin exposure. Learning how to mitigate your risks without avoiding everything you love, though, is not only possible but also empowering, as discussed in this chapter.

Chapter 5 Takeaways

- Buy organic for the items you eat most frequently or in the greatest quantities.
- Read ingredient lists carefully and avoid products that contain artificial sweeteners, colors, or preservatives, in addition to brominated vegetable oil, titanium dioxide, potassium bromate, or any other chemicals that you can't picture as a natural food.
- Buy food in bulk or in glass containers whenever possible to avoid harmful food packaging, and remember that paper packaging, while it may appear eco-friendly, can contain PFAS.
- If you must buy foods in plastic containers, remember the rhyme "5, 4, 1, and 2; all the rest are bad for you." These are the recycling codes found on products, and those numbered 5, 4, 1, and 2 are typically lower in chemicals.
- Buy certified GMO-free products if they contain corn or soy (and corn or soy by-products like cornstarch and soybean oil), two crops that are almost always genetically modified.
- Use your effort effectively by batch cooking, meal prepping, and enjoying leftovers of clean meals. For example, I make a dozen hard-boiled eggs every week or bake organic chicken breasts or wild-caught salmon fillets for use in several meals during the week.
- You don't have to throw out every food and drink that contains chemicals that happen to be in your kitchen and pantry right now. Commit instead to phasing in more "clean" foods over time and buying fewer products with problematic ingredients or packaging.
- Buy local or from farmers' markets whenever possible.

The food will be fresher, and because it's not meant to survive miles of travel or days on a store shelf, it often contains fewer synthetic chemicals; smaller companies are less likely to use these synthetic chemicals than larger manufacturers.

CHAPTER 6
What's Really in Your Personal-Care Products

FOR CENTURIES, WOMEN all over the world have been dying to be beautiful... literally. In China, women bound their feet for hundreds of years to appear more alluring to men, suffering spinal deformities, pelvic pain, posture problems, and difficulty walking as a result.[1] In Renaissance Europe and Victorian England, women applied extracts of deadly nightshade—a toxic plant known to paralyze and even kill—to whiten their skin or dilate their eyes to achieve a wide-eyed, breathless look, risking blurry vision and blindness for the effect.[2] During the eighteenth century, royalty and other high-society women wore foundation made with lead, sometimes developing lead poisoning as a result.[3] In the 1930s, French scientists popularized a skin cream made from radium and thorium—both radioactive elements—claiming the product would smooth unevenness and reverse aging.[4] In the United States, sixteen women became seriously injured or blinded in the 1930s after using Lash Lure, an eyelash dye made from paraphenylenediamine—a toxin still used in some hair dyes today.[5]

While these stories may sound shocking, not much has changed since then. Today, we still use cosmetics and personal-care products that have harmful effects, increasing the risk of everything from cancer to autoimmune disorders, disrupting hormone and immune function, making us more susceptible to allergic reactions, and even boosting our susceptibility to premature death. As proof, just look to the very public lawsuit against Johnson & Johnson, alleging the company knowingly sold baby powder contaminated with asbestos, which has been blamed for causing women to develop ovarian cancer (some plaintiffs have even died since the lawsuit began).[6] While this example may sound extreme, thousands of unregulated toxins exist in our cosmetics and personal-care products, and they're harming our health.

At the same time, we've seen a big boom in "clean" beauty and personal-care products, with retailers like Sephora and Target creating standards and logos to designate items that contain fewer synthetic ingredients. The only problem is that there are no universal standards or regulations for "clean" cosmetics and personal-care products, so what one company or retailer considers safe may not be truly safe or consistent with what is considered safe by other companies and retailers. That's why it pays to learn how to find authentically clean products.

Before we get to details, I want to share my journey to cleaner personal-care products because it was (and still is) a journey. And I've learned a lot along the way that can help you make smarter choices without sacrificing what you value or the way you want to look.

After I had my epiphany on my bathroom floor (see the Introduction), I knew I wanted an overhaul. I've never been much into makeup or the kind of person who has an intense skin or hair routine, but nearly everything I was using on my face, hair, skin, and nails contained toxic ingredients. Many of those toxic ingredients disrupt hormone function, interfere with immunity, and cause a host of other health problems. In short, I was dousing myself in a giant chemical cocktail every day, all in the name of "beauty" and "hygiene." And the irony of it all was that I didn't feel particularly beautiful or healthy putting all these toxins in, on, and around my skin, hair, and nails.

I didn't immediately throw out everything the day I decided to clean up my routine, though. I made slow, calculated choices over the course of years, starting with what seemed to me like the most obvious offenders: the products I slathered and lathered on in the shower every day. I began by trading conventional soap and my brand-name shampoo and conditioner for products that scored a 1 on the Environmental Working Group's Skin Deep database (see www.ewg.org/skindeep/). This free online database rates the safety of more than ninety-six thousand products on a scale from 1 to 10, with 10 indicating products and ingredients that are the most hazardous.

Next, I started to consider what I used in the greatest quantity on the largest surface of my body: my moisturizing lotion. This, for me, was a must-change, and while the earliest iterations of all-natural moisturizers didn't smell as good as the fruity stuff I was accustomed to using, I'm grateful I stopped rubbing chemicals on, in, and around the largest organ of my body (our skin!). In fact, the skin acts like such an effective sponge that many topical drugs are the most effective way to get medicine into our bodies.

Not every swap, though, was an instant or immediate success. When I first tried one brand of nontoxic face moisturizer, for example, I broke out, and it took days to get the product's ingredients, while all plant-based and nontoxic, out of my system. Here's the lesson: not all clean products may jibe with your skin or hair—a situation that is no different from conventional products made from synthetic (read: irritating) ingredients.

A similar situation happened when I first stopped using conventional antiperspirant, which has been associated (but not definitively linked) with an increased breast cancer risk (more on this on page 173).[7] I tried all the plant-based deodorants available in the early 2000s, but no matter which one I used, I still had to wear undershirts with built-in pads when I saw patients or I'd have pit stains or pools of perspiration right on the exam table! Since then, deodorant technology has improved substantially, and there's now a plethora of clean and effective options. I've also learned how to make my own DIY deodorant (recipe on page 175), which works just as well, if not better, than some store-bought brands. (I've also made DIY laundry detergent and cleaning products, and while my homemade products are just as effective as conventional versions and truly safe—and oftentimes cheaper—because I live an inordinately busy life, I now purchase safe, vetted deodorants and other products from progressive brands.)

If you're wondering why I made that sweaty sacrifice years ago when antiperspirants weren't (and still haven't been) proven to increase breast cancer risk, I'll tell you. While it's not conclusive, there's enough scientific evidence to suggest a relationship between antiperspirant use and increased breast cancer risk. I have a family history of the disease, so I didn't want to apply it to my armpits—a highly absorbent area with many sweat glands and lymph nodes, not to mention close proximity to breast tissue—only to have research catch up and conclude that antiperspirants may, in fact, increase the risk of breast cancer. This is the precautionary principle at its finest: *When an activity raises threats of harm to human health or the environment, precautionary measures should be taken, even if a cause-and-effect relationship has not been fully established scientifically.*[8]

This leads to another lesson I learned on my journey to achieve clean beauty: What you may initially think are sacrifices often turn out to be win-wins for both your health and your appearance. When I first switched to clean shampoo, for example, the products didn't work. My hair looked greasy, even if I had washed it that morning. But in a few weeks' time, my scalp adjusted, producing less oil. Now I don't have to wash my hair as frequently, and it's much less damaged and softer and healthier as a result. It also took me a long time to find and switch to a clean version of mascara that I really liked—before doing so, I simply limited how often I used conventional mascara. So, reducing your exposure can mean finding a clean product to replace a more toxic one; it can also mean changing your behavior so that you're simply not exposed to a toxin as often as you had been previously.

Today, I'm still looking for new or more effective ways to clean up my personal-care regime. For example, I recently decided to try to reduce the toxicity of getting manicures. At first, this seemed like an impossible feat, since there are so many noxious chemicals in nailcare. At the same time, I know these chemicals, even if I'm exposed infrequently, can have serious health effects.[9] But I also find going to the nail salon to be a relaxing experience that I enjoy. So, while I used to do it somewhat frequently, I now limit my visits to once every other month in an attempt to lower my overall exposure. I was then pleasantly surprised when I found a polish with a rating of 1—the lowest hazard ranking on the EWG's Skin Deep database—that was a mainstream brand available for just four dollars at a nearby pharmacy. Now, I take this polish with me every time I go to my nail salon, along with a polish remover that doesn't contain acetone, which is a liquid solvent shown to cause headaches, irritation, respiratory problems, and possible organ toxicity.[10] While acetone-free polish removers don't work nearly as well, this product will get the job done with a little extra elbow grease—and then neither I nor the nail tech is breathing in or absorbing the acetone. I also bring a nontoxic skin lotion to the nail salon instead of the typically noxious stuff they use for the leg massage, as I simply don't want to skip any massage!

On that note, I absolutely adore a good full-body massage. Sure, it's indulgent and relaxing, but also the therapy has been shown to improve sleep, circulation, and immune function while lowering blood pressure and inflammation level. But I don't understand why so many parlors and spas use chemical-based massage oils, which inevitably undo some of massage's medicinal benefits when a practitioner is repetitively rubbing a toxic substance into warm, absorbent, sponge-like skin for an extended duration of time.

When I first asked about this at my local spa, they swore their oil was all-natural, showing me the product, which did have a holistic-looking label. But when I looked up the product online, I saw it contained chemical fragrance, parabens, and a number of other toxins. I don't necessarily blame the spa for not knowing what was in their oil, as it's easy to be blindsided by "natural" products or those sold for holistic purposes. But the lesson here is that it pays to do your own research. A few years later, when I joined a large and popular massage service chain, I also discovered that their "organic" oil was misleading and mislabeled. I found a cleaner version on EWG's database that was also marketed for massage (so it wouldn't mess with my masseuse's skills) and started asking that my oil be used during our sessions.

It's important to stress that I haven't done everything I can to lower my toxic load when it comes to personal-care products. I've made the conscientious decision, for example, to continue to dye my hair blonde, at least for the time being. (I'm always a work in progress.) At the same time, I've learned how to extend the weeks between hair appointments, which (in another example of what may seem like a sacrifice at first) has made my hair stronger and healthier. I also bring my own nontoxic detangler to hair appointments to prevent an additional last application of chemical-based products.

SOME KEY LESSONS ON FINDING CLEAN PERSONAL-CARE PRODUCTS

Less is more. I guarantee you don't need to use as many products as you do today. Reducing the number of products you use is the easiest way to reduce your toxic load.

Clean = better beauty. You've heard the saying, "Beauty comes from the inside out," and the maxim couldn't be more accurate when it comes to nontoxic personal-care products: Using fewer chemicals on your body, face, hair, and nails will make them healthier, which in turn will cause them to look more radiant, nourished, and glowing.

Trial and error are key. If the all-natural deodorant or toothpaste you used a decade ago didn't work as well as you had hoped, try today's iterations. New technology and a proliferation of clean companies have made nontoxic products safer, more effective, better smelling, and easier to use. Clean personal-care products can also differ greatly from one to the other, so experiment with different brands and formulations to find the right one for you.

Don't let perfect be the enemy of good. There's no golden rule saying that once you go clean, you have to make every product swap possible. Use as many clean products as you can, but at the same time, know it's okay to make a conscientious decision to continue to use a certain conventional product or service.

Go slow. I didn't toss out my entire toiletry bag or cosmetics kit the day I decided to pay more attention to my personal-care regimen. Start by making one or two swaps, then when you run out of something, switch to a cleaner alternative.

Prioritize what you use the most and the most frequently. Scouring the web for clean eye shadow if you wear it only infrequently isn't as critical as swapping out the lotion you slather over your entire body twice daily. Get the biggest bang for your buck by updating the products you use daily in large quantities, like soap, body lotion, shampoo, toothpaste, and sunscreen. If you're female, prioritize using nontoxic deodorant and organic tampons or pads, since conventional versions may increase cancer risk (as discussed later in this chapter).

In the next few pages, you'll discover what's really in your personal-care products, what effects those conventional chemicals can have on your body, and how you can find and use safer and more effective products. Let's start.

Personal-Care Products: Tons of Toxins and Little Regulation

The average American woman uses twelve personal-care products daily, exposing herself to at least 168 unique chemicals every day.[11] These stats are worse for teens, with research showing that the average teenage girl uses seventeen personal-care products daily that contain a total of 174 unique chemicals.[12] While most people assume that whatever's in their soap, toothpaste, moisturizer, hair gel, and other personal-care products must be safe or else it wouldn't be sold, nothing could be further from the truth. Many chemicals in personal-care products have been linked to cancer, obesity, fertility problems, asthma, and learning and developmental disorders, among other health concerns.[13] Oftentimes, these toxins are both endocrine-disrupting chemicals (EDCs) and immune-disrupting chemicals (IDCs), interfering with hormone health and function while stoking the kind of inflammation that can lead to chronic disease.[14]

If you think there's no way your personal-care products could cause this much harm, since you're only dabbing a bit here or spraying a little there, studies show that the chemicals in cosmetics and other products can cause adverse health effects at "very low doses."[15] Although there's no exact way to measure a "very low dose," or to know how much exposure can or will cause harmful health effects, studies have shown that, for many chemicals, exposure as low as parts per trillion can show up in human blood and urine and create changes in the body.[16] In addition, many chemicals in personal-care products have been shown to get absorbed into the bloodstream[17]—one reason why people who use more personal-care products have higher levels of phthalates, parabens, and other common personal-care chemicals in their urine than those who use fewer such products.[18]

If our personal-care products are *this* toxic, why are they allowed to be used and sold? The answer, no pun intended, isn't pretty. More than ten thousand chemicals exist in American cosmetics and personal-care products, and only eleven have ever been banned by the US Food and Drug Administration (FDA). Compare that with the 1,400-plus chemicals banned from use in personal-care products in other countries.[19] One reason for this lack of oversight is that, up until recently, the FDA hasn't regulated chemicals in cosmetics and other personal-care products *at all*. For example, companies didn't have to register their products with the FDA, provide the agency with ingredient lists, adopt *good manufacturing practices* (GMPs), or even report adverse effects.[20] If a product did have obvious side effects or health concerns, the FDA didn't even have the authority to recall it.[21]

This changed somewhat in 2022, when President Biden signed into law the Modernization of Cosmetics Regulation Act, which mandates companies register products with the FDA, report adverse effects within fifteen days (whether consumers actually report adverse effects to companies is another matter altogether), disclose allergens in fragrance ingredients, and follow GMPs. The FDA can also now recall products if it believes they endanger the public's safety. But the law, while a step in the right direction, doesn't give the FDA the power to review, restrict, or ban any chemicals used in personal-care products.[22] This means that companies can continue to use toxins, including known carcinogens, in their personal-care products.

The Price of Beauty: What Personal-Care Chemicals Can Do to the Body

If you've ever had acne, rosacea, hives, or any other dermatological issue, you may not think that your skin is incredible, but it is—and not just because it looks good. The biggest organ in the body, the skin is highly complex, with one square inch packing 19 million cells, 1,000 nerve ends, 650 sweat glands, and 20 blood vessels[23] into a stack of cells 2 millimeters thick—that's about the thickness of a book cover.[24]

While the skin is one of many wonders of the human body, it's also highly absorbent. This isn't great news if you expose it to dozens, if not hundreds, of chemicals daily. In fact, the skin can absorb up to 64 percent of the contaminants in water (another reason to filter your shower water—see page 113).[25] Many of these absorbed contaminants can then enter the bloodstream, giving them the ability to travel to cells, tissues, and organs throughout the body.

Adding insult to injury, many products have added chemicals known as penetration or permeation enhancers, which are used to increase the skin's absorption of the item's ingredients. Permeation enhancers are often added to products for softening the deeper layers of the skin, carrying medicine to muscles or joints, or even entering the bloodstream for systemic effects (like transdermal patches, which are more likely used for medicinal purposes like calming seasickness than for personal care). But these enhancers are not safe in most instances, especially if used for long periods of time. (In some cases, however, the benefits of the medication may outweigh the risks, which is why it's always advisable to speak with a doctor before taking these meds or making any changes to your current routine.) These noxious chemicals work by impairing the epidermal barrier so they can enter the skin more easily, bringing other toxins into the body with them.[26] Whatever we rub, soak, spray, or lather into our hair can be absorbed by our scalp, which is part of our skin. In fact, the scalp is more absorbent than most other areas of the body because it is packed with blood vessels that supply quickly growing hair follicles, and that also speeds absorption.[27]

All these facts become more disconcerting when you examine exactly what's in your personal-care products. Remember that idea of mixture toxicity in relation to food, discussed on page 145? Yep, that applies to personal-care products, too. While there are hundreds of possible chemicals and chemical combinations used in personal-care products, the following are nine of the most toxic ones, according to the EWG.[28] Note that you will find some but not all these ingredients listed on the products' labels, which is why it pays to check the products on a third-party website or app, like the EWG's Skin Deep database:

Formaldehyde: a known carcinogen, used in color cosmetics, hair straighteners, hair gel, body wash and soap, baby shampoo, and other products.

Paraformaldehyde: a type of formaldehyde, used in a range of products.

Methylene glycol: a type of formaldehyde, used in a range of products.

Quaternium-15: a toxin that releases formaldehyde, used in a range of products, including hair conditioners and other styling products, body lotions, and body cleaners.

Mercury: a toxic heavy metal linked to kidney and nervous system damage, used in skin-lightening creams, anti-aging creams, antiseptic soaps, and other products.

Dibutyl and diethylhexyl phthalates: endocrine disruptors linked to reproductive harm, used in color cosmetics, lotions, body washes, hair-care products, nail polishes, and other products.

Isobutyl and isopropyl parabens: endocrine-disrupting parabens linked to cancer and reproductive harm, used in shampoos, conditioners, lotions, face cleansers, and other products.

Per- and polyfluoroalkyl (PFAS) substances: the "forever chemicals" linked to cancer, in long-lasting lipsticks, mascaras, foundations, and other products.

Coal tar like m- and o-phenylenediamine: chemicals linked to cancer and DNA damage, used in hair dyes and other products (the same product found in Lash Lure that blinded women in the 1930s).

A handful of states like California and Maryland have already banned from personal-care products some of these chemicals. What's more, they have also banned the following additional chemicals. Note that most of these provisions go into effect in 2025:[29]

Butylated hydroxyanisole (BHA): a synthetic preservative linked to cancer and reproductive harm, used in lipsticks, eyeliners, moisturizers, and other products, including food products.

Diethanolamine (DEA): a chemical that reacts with other compounds to form a "reasonably anticipated" human carcinogen, used in creamy or foamy products like shampoos and shaving creams.

Fragrance or perfume: a vague term that usually means a product includes hundreds of unknown chemicals (but typically phthalates) from more than 3,600 toxins, used to make scents; some are linked to cancer, reproductive harm, immune disruption, and organ toxicity.

Toluene: a colorless liquid linked to nervous system damage and decreased immunity, used in nail polishes, hair dyes, and other products.

Triclosan and triclocarban: antimicrobial compounds linked to thyroid interference and microbiome harm, used in toothpastes, deodorants, and hand sanitizers, in addition to other products like plastic cutting boards and cookware; they have been banned by the FDA for use in soaps and body washes.

Talc: a natural mineral linked to cancer that may also contain asbestos, used in eye shadows, blotting sheets, baby powders, and deodorants.

Polyethylene glycols (PEGS): chemicals linked to cancer that thicken products and speed skin absorption (permeation enhancers), used in soaps, makeup, creams, and other products.

THE BEAUTY INDUSTRY'S UGLY TRUTH

Women of color, especially Black women, tend to use more toxic personal-care products and have higher detectable levels of beauty-based chemicals in their urine and blood than do white women.[30] One reason for this is that women of color, in an attempt to conform to unfair Caucasian beauty standards, are more likely to use skin-lightening creams, hair relaxers, hair straighteners, vaginal douches, talc-based body powders, and other scented feminine-care products, all which have been linked to reproductive harm and cancer.[31] Black women, in particular, buy nine times more hair-care products than any other demographic.[32]

The type of products marketed to women of color also contain more toxic chemicals, according to the research. One study found that 65 percent of all personal-care products on store shelves where women of color are more likely to shop contain chemicals of concern, like parabens, formaldehyde releasers, and unidentified fragrances.[33]

The net effect of this, unfortunately, is markedly higher rates of cancer, particularly breast cancer, among women of color. Black women who regularly dye their hair with a permanent dye have a 44 to 75 percent greater chance of developing breast cancer, while those who use chemical straighteners are 30 percent more likely to develop the disease than women of other demographics.[34] Black women are also more likely in general to be diagnosed with breast cancer before the age of fifty, they develop more aggressive subtypes, and they die more often from the disease, compared to other demographics.[35]

If you're a woman of color, resist the racist sociocultural standards and use fewer products overall, while paying closer attention to those products that remain in your beauty regimen; choose products that have been vetted for safety. If you lighten your skin or straighten or relax your hair, consider giving up these habits.

Health *and* Beauty: How to Find Cleaner Cosmetics and Personal-Care Products without Compromise

If you've ever looked at a product's ingredient list, you probably have felt like you need a chemistry degree to understand and decipher all the multisyllabic, confusing chemical names. Similar to how sugar can hide in foods under dozens of different names (maltodextrin, maltose, brown rice syrup, etc.), so can common chemicals in personal-care products. There are at least a dozen different names for formaldehyde, for example, as well as its carcinogenic cousins, a class of compounds that release formaldehyde when broken down.[36] Also, just like with food, seeing the words *natural*, *clean*, or *nontoxic* on personal-care products doesn't mean they are free of harmful ingredients, since none of these terms are regulated by the FDA.[37] And since the FDA considers the chemical makeup of "fragrance" in personal-care products to be a trade secret (along with certain food formulas, like that for Coca-Cola), seeing the term on an ingredient list provides no context: it could encompass hundreds of unknown chemicals.

As consumers, we are blinded to what's really in the products we use, and manufacturers in the United States are given priority over the protection of human health. For these reasons, I show my patients and the high-school students to whom I give presentations how to scrutinize their favorite products using the EWG's Skin Deep database. The online site, which you can also access through the EWG's catchall app Healthy Living, allows you to enter a product name in the search bar or scan its barcode to find its ranking from 1 to 10. On the database, rankings 1 and 2 indicate low hazard, 3 to 6 are moderate hazard, and 7 to 10 are high hazard. I recommend avoiding all products rated anywhere over 2.

While there are other databases for this information, like Think

Dirty, Clearya, and Yuka, EWG's Skin Deep database is among the most scientific and comprehensive. If there's not enough data on a specific ingredient to rank it properly, the database reflects that in the item's score. However, if you already use an app that you like and know it's an independent (meaning not company-funded) and trusted source, continue to use it. The message here is simply to start analyzing those products as often and in any way you can.

In addition to using a clean product website or app, here are seven best practices to develop a safer personal-care regimen:

Use fewer products overall. I repeat this because it's critical: the fewer products you use, the fewer you'll need and the lower your chemical exposure will be for the rest of your life. This is especially important if you're pregnant or nursing, as studies show that the chemicals in personal-care products can be absorbed by a growing fetus, as well as transfer into children through breast milk.[38]

Avoid labels using the word *fragrance*. This usage can mean hundreds of undisclosed toxins. If you like scented products, look for those that use natural essential oils, tree resins, and other botanical extracts, which can be safe. Some perfumes and fragrances may also be marketed as clean; just be sure to suss them out using the Skin Deep database or other clean beauty app.

Head to the kitchen. This is the way to have truly clean personal-care products. Use almond or jojoba oil as a makeup remover; coconut oil as a body moisturizer, shaving cream, or hair conditioner; brown sugar or coffee grounds to exfoliate skin; brewed coffee to relieve eye puffiness; baking soda mixed with water as a toothpaste or facial cleanser; lemon or lemon oil to reduce age spots; topical yogurt as an anti-aging treatment. The list goes on. Look online for specific measurements and more ideas (and check out my recipe for DIY deodorant on page 175).

Choose phthalate-, paraben-, and fragrance-free products. While seeing these claims on a personal-care product doesn't guarantee it won't contain other harmful toxins, you'll at least reduce your exposure to these particular noxious babies. For example, simply choosing sulfate-free mainstream hair products can lower the toxicity score on the EWG's database from a 5 or 6 to a 4—that's not perfect, but it's certainly better.

Opt for USDA-certified organic skincare. This means a product's ingredients come from plants that were organically grown. Otherwise, seeing simply the word *organic* on the label can mean it has a few organic ingredients, but may also mean it includes harmful toxins.

Look for "EWG Verified" or "Cosmos Standards." These are third-party certifications that indicate safe products. In the instance of the EWG, its verified products don't contain any "unacceptable" chemicals of concern—a list that includes several hundred toxins—while meeting all the nonprofit's standards for ingredient disclosure and naming, including the ingredients in "fragrance." Whole Foods Market also has fairly strict guidelines for the types of personal-care products they accept, based on chemical inclusion. And some big-box stores like Target and Sephora offer clean lines that meet their proprietary safety standards; even so, it's best to double-check these products using a clean product app or website.[39]

Avoid the ingredients listed on pages 164–66. Also avoid those that contain penetration or permeation enhancers, like isopropyl and propylene glycol, and any ingredient that starts with the prefix *peg*, which is short for *pegylated*.[40]

Here are other considerations for using specific personal-care products:

SUNSCREENS

Most sunscreens are "chemical" sunscreens, which means they block the sun's rays by using chemicals that get absorbed into the skin, where they work to negate the effect of those harmful rays. The problem with these products, however, is that they're highly toxic, as you may imagine. In 2019, the FDA, which regulates sunscreens as an over-the-counter drug, stated that only two active ingredients in sunscreen—zinc oxide and titanium dioxide—could be considered safe. The rest are now under FDA investigation, including the common chemical ingredients oxybenzone and avobenzone, along with cinoxate, dioxybenzone, ensulizole, homosalate, meradimate, octinoxate, octisalate, octocrylene, padimate O, and sulisobenzone.

Zinc oxide and titanium dioxide are often the active (and only) ingredients in "physical" or "mineral" sunscreens, which block harmful rays by forming a physical layer on the skin, meaning they are not absorbed the way chemical sunscreens are.[41] Among these two mineral sunscreens, I opt for zinc oxide, after recent studies on titanium dioxide in food found health risks that may or may not be extrapolated to skin absorption.[42] While some mineral sunscreens leave a whitish film, the products do vary, so try different brands until you find one that works for you.

No matter what sunscreen you use, even if it's a conventional product, never skip using the sunscreen, especially between the hours of 10 a.m. and 2 p.m., when the sun's rays are strongest. Cover all areas of the skin, and don't forget your ears and toes. Exposing yourself to UV radiation from the sun can cause DNA damage that leads to premature aging and several types of skin cancer, including basal cell carcinoma, the most common form of the disease, affecting one in five Americans by age seventy. Having five or more sunburns doubles the risk of developing melanoma,[43] which is why always wearing sunscreen is critical, no matter what it's made of. In short, wearing a chemical sunscreen is better than wearing nothing at all.

LIPSTICKS

Even expensive lipsticks can contain lead and mercury, two heavy metals that can be more toxic when ingested, as most people do when they wear lipstick.[44] Instead, look for mineral-based products that are EWG Verified.

TAMPONS AND OTHER FEMININE-CARE PRODUCTS

A woman's vaginal canal is more permeable than any other area of her body, and she can absorb chemicals and drugs quickly through her vagina—up to ten times faster than if she swallowed a pill containing the same ingredients.[45] That's a problem, since many tampons, pads, and other feminine-care products contain phthalates, parabens, heavy metals, fragrance, plastic, antimicrobials and other pesticides, and volatile organic compounds (VOCs), some of which are potential carcinogens.[46] And manufacturers of feminine-care products aren't doing enough to ensure the safety of these products. One study found elevated levels of heavy metals in thirty tampons from fourteen different brands, with levels of lead higher in nonorganic brands than in organic brands.[47] This is why I recommend buying only 100 percent cotton tampons, pads, and feminine-care products. If they are affordable for you, look for tampons and pads made from 100 percent USDA- or GOTS (Global Organic Textile Standard) certified organic cotton; otherwise, the term "organic" can mean the product contains a few organic ingredients along with potential toxins.

In recent years, period underwear—with built-in padding designed to absorb blood and fluid—has become more popular, but some of these products can contain toxic PFAS and toxic dyes; check the labels and marketing materials, and shop for those that state they don't include these chemicals. If you prefer to use menstrual cups, look for products made with 100 percent silicone, which is the only plastic material generally considered safe for products that come into contact with sensitive tissue, such as the cervix and vaginal canal.

HAIRSPRAYS AND DRY SHAMPOOS

Aerosolized products like hairspray and dry shampoo, along with antiperspirants and deodorants, increase your risk of chemical exposure through inhalation and skin absorption. Look for pump-spray products that are rated "low hazard" on the Skin Deep database and are free of fragrances, formaldehyde, and other chemicals.

ANTIPERSPIRANTS AND DEODORANTS

Just like the genital area, the underarm area is highly absorbent, with a ton of sweat glands and lymph nodes (small clusters of immune cells that filter foreign substances), which are in close proximity to breast tissue. For these reasons, what you spray, roll, or apply to this area can be critical to your overall breast health. Antiperspirants, but not deodorants, can contain aluminum compounds small enough to be absorbed by the sweat glands. These aluminum compounds can also accumulate in breast tissue[48] and are a risk factor for breast cancer, according to some studies.[49] While the American Cancer Society says the link between aluminum in antiperspirants and breast cancer isn't clear, I remind you of the precautionary principle: better safe than sorry.[50] In addition, both antiperspirant and conventional deodorant can contain synthetic fragrance, parabens, and harmful antimicrobial agents like triclosan, which don't belong in our bodies. For these reasons, forgo antiperspirants and opt for an EWG Verified deodorant, many which contain natural ingredients like baking soda, tapioca, or arrowroot starch to prevent sweating.

NAILS AND MANI/PEDIS

Bring your own nontoxic base coat and research other products that don't contain toxic chemicals such as toluene, dibutyl phthalate, TPHP, xylene, ethyl tosylamide, camphor, formaldehyde, formaldehyde resin, and parabens. Surprisingly, I found a few popular base coats at my local chain pharmacy store that were rated 1 or 2 on the EWG's Skin Deep database.

MAKEUP REMOVERS

Use a nontoxic oil, such as almond oil or coconut oil, making sure not to get it in your eyes. Pure oils like these, without added perfume or fragrance, can readily remove a variety of cosmetics, such as foundation and mascara.

DIY DEODORANT THAT WORKS

This deodorant, made from ingredients you likely have in your kitchen or medicine cabinet, has no toxins and works just as well, if not better, than many chemical-free brands on store shelves, without leaving any white residue (although be careful when wearing thin blouses or silk, which can absorb stains from the oil-based ingredients). One batch takes only ten minutes to make and can last up to four months. Just be sure to store it in a cool, dry place, as coconut oil can melt in temperatures greater than 75ºF.

2½ teaspoons unrefined coconut oil
2½ teaspoons unrefined shea butter
2 teaspoons baking soda
½ cup arrowroot
6 drops lavender or orange essential oil
6 drops grapefruit essential oil
2 drops tea tree oil

Place coconut oil and shea butter in a glass bowl or jar, then place the jar in a medium saucepan. Add enough water to the saucepan to surround the bowl or jar, then bring the water to a boil over medium heat.

Stir the melted coconut oil and shea butter, then stir in the baking soda, arrowroot, and essential oils.

Transfer the mixture to a small glass jar with a lid and allow to cool at room temperature. Once cooled, cover with the lid and set aside until ready to use. Apply with your fingertips.

DETOXIFY

We all use personal-care products every day, but thankfully it's now easy, convenient, and sometimes less expensive to choose items made without noxious chemicals. If you haven't experimented with clean personal-care products in a while, give them a chance, since ingredient efficacy and product technology have come a long way in recent years. These alternative products can be just as good, if not better, than conventional chemical-based items.

Chapter 6 Takeaways

- You don't have to throw out all your soap, lotions, cosmetics, hair products, and personal-care products today. When you finish something, replace it with a cleaner alternative that you have chosen using a trusted database like the EWG's Skin Deep.
- Be patient when using new clean products. Your skin or hair may need a few days or even weeks to adapt to the new product, which may not be as harsh as what you're used to—meaning it doesn't remove as much oil, sweat, and other natural substances as conventional products might.
- Take a hard look at your morning and evening skincare and hygiene routine. Do you really need to use all the products you do? I've found that less is more when it comes to personal-care products, and using fewer can often allow those you do use to work more effectively.
- Scan and shop! If you download the EWG's Healthy Living app, you can simply scan the barcode of products you're considering and get the nonprofit's opinion on how clean it is. You can also type the product's name into the EWG's Skin Deep database website to obtain the rating.
- Consider bringing your own safe products to a hair or nail salon, which is what I do every time I get my nails done, bringing my own base coat, polish, and acetone-free polish remover; similarly, I bring my own detangler whenever I get my hair cut or highlighted. You can simply tell your stylist or technician that you have sensitive skin and know these products you've brought don't contain anything that will irritate it.

CHAPTER 7
What's Really Inside Your Home

WHEN I FIRST realized just how dangerous environmental chemicals can be, the rose-colored glasses I had been wearing for my entire life—the same metaphorical glasses that prevent most of us from recognizing how many toxins we encounter—suddenly fell off. What I was left with was a new way of seeing the world—one that, once seen, I couldn't unsee. This new vision led me everywhere, including where and whenever I traveled.

A few years ago, for example, I traveled to Costa Rica with my family for the first time. It's a spectacular country, particularly the Nicoya Peninsula. This is a designated Blue Zone, one of only five places in the world with the largest population of centenarians—people who live to one hundred years or older—thanks in part to a low incidence of lifestyle diseases like cancer, Alzheimer's, diabetes, and obesity.[1] There are many reasons why Nicoya is a Blue Zone, including that this rural peninsula is far from cities, industrial manufacturers, and fast-food chains, with almost as many horses as cars and few sources of immediate pollution. Much of what residents eat in Nicoya is locally grown, with little packaging, processing, or pesticides; and to get around, you have to walk almost everywhere, oftentimes over hilly terrain.

Yet amid all this low-toxin living, I was disappointed—although not surprised—to be reminded of how Westerners live when my family and I walked into our hotel. From the moment we entered the lobby, I could smell the carpet deodorizer, window cleaner, bleach, air freshener, and insecticide that covered the hotel's halls, walls, countertops, and corridors. I don't have a particularly sensitive nose—quite the opposite, which is why I used to love those overpowering plug-in air fresheners—but the contrast when it comes to daily chemical exposure was eye-opening.

Don't get me wrong: I appreciate a clean hotel just as much as anyone else. But there are plenty of ways to clean, as you'll discover in this chapter, that don't make our environment "dirty" with toxic air. This isn't just me being reactionary; the air inside our homes, offices, and other indoor spaces can be two to five times more polluted than the outside air, according to the Environmental Protection Agency (EPA). And this is true even if you live in a large, industrialized city.[2] The reason? Nearly every home good we own—including furniture, bedding, carpeting, cleaning supplies, window treatments, flooring, air fresheners, dry-cleaned clothing, and electronics—emits chemicals that end up in our air, our dust, and ultimately, our bodies. As a result, indoor air pollution can increase the risk of developing serious health effects, like cancer, neurological disorders, and endocrine and immune system damage.[3]

While there's not much we can do about the air inside hotels, offices, theaters, and other public places, except to suggest to lobby management that they prioritize green cleaning products and lower-emission paint and furniture, there are dozens of simple steps you can take to drastically improve the air quality inside your home. Thankfully, these steps don't include throwing out everything you own or never touching a chemical-based cleaner again. As I learned after years of trial, tribulation, and, most important, lots of research, making simple changes to how you clean and what your furniture is made of can significantly reduce your exposure to indoor air pollution. Making these simple changes will help you turn your home into the safe space and the sanctuary many of us believe it to be.

The Price of Conventional Clean: Chemicals in Cleaning Products

For many, the easiest starting place for reducing indoor air pollution is to rethink how you clean your home—which is exactly what I did after that epiphany on my bathroom floor fifteen years ago. While I used to be fanatical about disinfecting every surface, believing that I was protecting my young children from dangerous germs by doing so, I quickly realized I was exposing them to much more harmful substances by using chemicals strong enough to wipe out most good microbes, too. After all, that's what makes disinfectant a disinfectant or product that kills bacteria—both the "bad" kind like salmonella and *E. coli* and the "good" kind that help fortify our microbiome. Common disinfectants include bleach and all-purpose cleaners, and they are often marketed to kill "99.9 percent of germs."

By comparison, cleaning with water and soap made from castile (a combination of vegetable oils) or other natural oils (like those found in Dr. Bronner's soap) is effective in limiting germs without exposing you and your family to harsh disinfectants. Cleaning with soap and water is what I do for almost all instances in my home, and it's how environmental health experts recommend everyone clean almost everything—especially in the wake of the Covid-19 pandemic, when our collective use of disinfecting products skyrocketed.[4] During the pandemic, researchers found that the more often people used disinfectants, the higher levels they had of harmful chemical compounds in their blood and breast milk.[5] These compounds can interfere with the health of the body's microbiome. They can even cause weight gain in children who live in homes where there's high disinfectant use, making them obesogens.[6] (As a reminder, *obesogens* are chemicals that disrupt metabolic health and affect fat cell development, storage, and size.)

But it's not just disinfectants that are inherently harmful. Conventional dishwasher and laundry detergents; soap scum, mold, and mildew removers; window, grout, tile, kitchen, and carpet cleaners; air fresheners, fabric softeners, and deodorizers; insecticides, rodenticides, and other pesticides; and floor, car, and wood polishes—basically every traditional cleaning product can contain chemicals harmful to human health. While most people assume that cleaning regularly with modern-day products makes for a healthier home, research shows the opposite, with one Norwegian study finding that prolonged use of chemical-based cleaning supplies may be as bad for our health as smoking.[7]

While that's a shocking stat, the reality could be worse, since no one really knows what exactly is in conventional cleaning products, including the US government. While the Consumer Product Safety Commission—an independent federal agency that regulates consumer products, including household cleaners—requires manufacturers to list "chemicals of known concern," most chemicals used have never been tested for safety—meaning they can't be chemicals of known concern because we don't technically know enough about them.[8] In fact, of the tens of thousands of chemicals registered for use in the United States, only 1 percent have ever undergone safety testing.[9]

What we do know, though, is that many chemicals used in cleaning products are both endocrine-disrupting chemicals (EDCs) and immune-disrupting chemicals (IDCs) that, even in low doses, can cause adverse health effects like rashes, asthma, and allergic reactions, in addition to inflammation of the immune system over time and with regular exposure.[10] Quaternary ammonium compounds (QACs), or "quats," commonly used in disinfectants, antiseptics, and detergents, have been found to increase the risk of asthma and skin irritation.[11] Some EDCs in cleaning products, of which there are too many to list, may interfere with hormone health in amounts as small as one part per trillion—the equivalent of one drop of water diluted in twenty Olympic-size swimming pools.[12] And because of that phenomenon known as mixture toxicity—when chemicals combine to produce more harmful substances than individual toxins themselves—no level of exposure to conventional cleaners may be safe. What's more, chemicals in cleaning products often stay on those surfaces or fall to the ground, where they can stick to toys and other objects, then be picked up by children and pets through hand-to-mouth or paw-to-mouth contact.

What kind of health problems have been associated with cleaning products? According to the Environmental Working Group, 53 percent of household cleaners contain ingredients like bleach, fragrance, and solvent chemicals that can harm the lungs, while 22 percent contain ingredients shown to trigger asthma in healthy people.[13] Some cleaning products can also contain formaldehyde, a known carcinogen; others include 1,4-dioxin or phthalates, which are suspected carcinogens. Products that contain bleach can also create carcinogenic fumes when exposed to other substances.[14] In addition to cancer and respiratory issues, many chemicals found in cleaning products have been shown to interfere with reproductive health and fertility or cause developmental problems in children—the latter being why women who work as household cleaners have one of the highest occupational risks of having children with birth defects.[15] Products that contain quaternary ammonium compounds can increase the risk for respiratory illness, exacerbate asthma, and possibly lead to long-term lung damage and conditions like chronic obstructive pulmonary disease (COPD).[16]

Unfortunately, even products marketed as "natural" or "green" can contain chemicals of concern, as these terms aren't regulated by the government and are used liberally at the manufacturer's discretion.[17] Clorox Green Works laundry detergent, for example, contains ingredients of high health hazard, according to the EWG—why the nonprofit gave it an F grade on its Guide to Healthy Cleaning database.[18] (The EWG's guide to Healthy Cleaning is similar to its Skin Deep database for personal-care products, but products are graded with letter scores ranging from A to F, with F being the worst or most hazardous. More than two thousand products have been scored using a rigorous methodology that considers the strength and severity of an association between an ingredient and a health outcome, as well as the credibility of the organization that conducted the research, while also pooling other databases created by academic institutions, government agencies, and independent panels.[19])

Here's another example. Whole Foods 365 Everyday Value unscented 2x concentrated liquid laundry detergent scored an F on the EWG's database because it contains sodium borate, an EDC linked to reproductive and developmental harm, along with other potentially harmful ingredients.[20]

At the same time, there *are* green cleaners that are truly nontoxic and that work just as well as conventional cleaning supplies. Studies even show that some nontoxic brands can disinfect and kill *E. coli* and the bacteria responsible for staph infections just as well as bleach.[21]

How to Clean Safely

While many cleaning products create more health hazards than they solve, it's possible to keep a clean house that's nontoxic—and I've done it for years. Here are my top tips that can help you reduce indoor air pollution while making your home a safer space:

Consult the EWG's Guide to Healthy Cleaning before buying. In the last chapter, you learned about the EWG's Skin Deep database, which is an incredible resource to identify nontoxic personal-care products. The nonprofit also makes a database for cleaning products, which you can download to your phone as part of its Healthy Living app or access through the EWG's website. Either way, the guide gives letter grades (A to F) for different categories of household cleaners, with an A indicating low toxicity and an F indicating high toxicity or little to no ingredient disclosure.[22] I recommend buying only A-graded items or those marked as EWG Verified, which is the organization's gold standard for nontoxic products.

Only "USDA-Certified Organic" has meaning. I've said it before, and it also applies to household cleaners: the word *organic* has no meaning unless it comes with the USDA-certified organic label, which guarantees at least 95 percent of a cleaning product's ingredients are derived from organically grown plants. (The ingredients for products with a 100% USDA-certified organic label derive entirely from organically grown plants).

DIY cleaners are just as effective as chemical cleaners. I can personally attest to this, as can *Good Housekeeping*, the magazine that's an authority on all things home economy.[23] DIY cleaners may require a little more elbow grease, but the payoff for your health is huge. As an added bonus, DIY household cleaners can be less expensive than conventional cleaning products, especially since you may already have many of the ingredients in your kitchen. Here are some DIY cleaning ingredients; for specific measurements and additional uses, see the recipes in Appendix 3 and look online for more ideas:

Lemon juice cuts grease and mineral buildup while acting as a natural bleach to whiten surfaces. Use it to remove stains from coffee pots and tea kettles, degrease stovetops and other surfaces, clean glass (when mixed with water), bleach clothing (when mixed with water), eliminate fridge odors, and wipe up stains from laminate countertops.

Baking soda absorbs odors and is mildly abrasive, making it ideal for scrubbing toilets, sinks, baths, and showers. You can also use it to clean bathroom drains, degrease dishes, polish kitchen appliances and utensils (when mixed with hydrogen peroxide), deodorize your fridge, and clean your oven (when mixed with water, then sprayed with vinegar).

White vinegar is the ultimate do-it-all cleaner, capable of removing soap scum and grease while deodorizing and disinfecting. Mix with water to clean windows, floors, kitchen countertops, toilets, the inside of your microwave, wine glasses, pots and pans, and any other surface or appliance you want to sparkle. You can also add vinegar to an empty dishwasher or coffee pot and run through one cycle to clean.

Castile soap cuts grease and dirt while working as a multipurpose cleaner. Mix with water to use as an all-purpose spray, floor cleaner, insect repellent, fruit and vegetable wash, or dog or cat shampoo.

Club soda removes stains from clothing, carpets, and furniture—just spray, blot, and repeat. You can also use it to clean windows, stainless steel pots, and cast-iron pans.

Coarse salt can be used to scrub clean greasy pans, coffee makers, and cloudy vases and glasses.

Upgrade your tool set. Having effective accessories can make cleaning a lot easier, reducing the need for harsh cleaners. Invest in a high-quality microfiber mop, squeegee for your shower, abrasive sponge for your kitchen and bathroom, and microfiber duster for your living areas and bedrooms. Rent or buy a steam cleaner to clean tile floors, countertops, upholstery, mattresses, appliances, and even shower grout (just be sure to avoid using any chemical cleaners that may come with the appliance). A good plunger or flexible metal snake is great to help unclog drains instead of using harsh drain chemicals that feed into our water system.

Don't fall for antibacterial or antimicrobial products. Avoid detergents, dishwashing liquids, vacuum cleaners, and any other products marketed as antibacterial, antimicrobial, or that contain triclosan, an antibacterial chemical banned by the FDA for use in liquid soap but still allowed in other items, including personal-care products, cosmetics, cutting boards, yoga mats, bathroom tile sealant, and some cleaning supplies and appliances. Exposure to triclosan and other synthetic antibacterial/microbial ingredients, including Microban (a brand-name antimicrobial), can trigger antibiotic resistance, making you more susceptible to untreatable infections. Adding insult to injury, antibacterial soap doesn't even prevent infectious illness any better than regular soap.[24]

If you want to use hand sanitizer, skip the store-bought stuff and opt instead for rubbing alcohol, also known as isopropyl alcohol, which you can find at any pharmacy or big-box store. Look for 70 percent isopropyl alcohol and make sure the product's inactive ingredients list only water. Fill a spray bottle with the alcohol and use the spray on your hands—the product works just like hand sanitizer, evaporating quickly, so you don't need tissues or towels. I like to fill a three-ounce travel spray bottle with rubbing alcohol and carry in my bag everywhere I go.

Avoid air fresheners, scented candles, carpet powders, and other deodorizers. They may smell nice, but these products are essentially inhalable chemicals, many which have been linked to cancer and nervous system damage. Conventional cleaners with a citrus or pine scent can emit terpenes—toxins that react with ozone in the air to form formaldehyde, a known carcinogen.[25] If you really want to scent your home, opt for candles made only from natural wax like soy, palm, or beeswax (as opposed to paraffin, which is often derived from petroleum) and that rely on 100 percent organic essential oils for fragrance.

Don't use "-cides." Pesticides like insecticides, rodenticides, fungicides, and termiticides are formulated to kill—that's what the suffix *cide* means. When I began evaluating the toxins in my home, I realized we had a literal war chest of things designed to kill creatures. That's a huge problem, according to the EPA, which calls home pesticides "inherently toxic," capable of increasing the risk of cancer while harming our endocrine, immune, and nervous systems and causing kidney and liver damage. As per the EPA, 80 percent of our pesticide exposure comes from use inside our homes, with some houses having measurable levels of up to a dozen pesticides at a time.[26] The solution? Seal small cracks and openings where pests can enter, vacuum often, and don't leave out food, pet food, or trash, which can attract pests. Depending on which kind of pest problem you have, non-kill traps or essential oils like tea tree may be an option. If your problem persists, talk with an expert about natural or low-toxic alternatives, which can include mechanical rodent traps that use catch-and-release or apply natural substances like peppermint oil and cayenne around your home to help deter pests. Explain to the professional that you don't want to use any industrial chemicals in your home owing to health reasons and ask if they can explain the different options before they apply any solution so that you can feel comfortable with the alternative.

Prioritize getting rid of household dust. Dust contributes significantly to indoor air pollution by trapping volatile organic compounds (VOCs) and other chemicals that can be given off by furniture and other home items. To get rid of dust, invest in a vacuum with a HEPA filter, which is more effective at picking up small particles, and use damp microfiber mops and dust cloths to clean other areas. A forced-air heating and cooling system that comes with high-quality filters can also help limit dust, but avoid ozone air purifiers, which can irritate your lungs without removing dust or other airborne particles, according to the EWG.[27]

Homesick: How Our Houses and the Things We Own Can Make Us Ill

Hundreds of chemicals in the products we own contribute to indoor air pollution. Many of these chemicals belong to a class of harmful substances known as *volatile organic compounds* (VOCs), which can migrate out of those products and "off-gas," meaning they are released into the air. It doesn't make a difference whether you can detect a chemical smell; even air that doesn't have any smell can be harmful. In other words, chemicals are often deceiving. And if you live in a big city, being more vigilant about toxins and making the following changes when possible is even more critical, since you're already exposed to more outdoor and, by proxy, indoor air pollutants.

Some home goods now contain labels or marketing information that state they're low- or no-VOC, meaning they emit only low levels of the harmful compounds or none at all. While looking for these labels is key, it's not always foolproof, which is why it pays to know something about the most common VOCs. The more you know, the easier they'll be to avoid. Here's a breakdown:

Flame retardants are found in upholstered furniture, pillows, carpets, electronics, baby products, and other home goods. Flame retardants are chemicals intentionally added to products to help limit their flammability. While this may sound like a good thing, flame retardants may increase the risk of cancer, thyroid disruption, infertility, developmental problems, and low IQ in children, among other health problems.[28]

In 1975, California passed a law requiring manufacturers to include flame retardants in furniture and other home goods to give people more time to escape a burning home. Because companies didn't want to make special products for sale only in the state of California, they started to infuse all home goods with the chemicals. Even though the law was rescinded in 2013, and the use of polybrominated diphenyl ethers (PBDEs)—the most common flame retardant ingredient—was phased out, some electronics, clothing, baby products, and car seats, along with older upholstered furniture, carpets, and other home goods, still contain the chemicals.[29] In addition, manufacturers have started using "regrettable substitutes"—similar chemical compounds that are just as harmful—in lieu of PBDEs, notably brominated flame retardants, or bromophenols, which have been linked to hormone disruption, fertility issues, and learning problems in children. A recent study found bromophenols present in 88 percent of breast milk samples,[30] while older studies have found detectable levels of PBDEs in 97 percent of Americans' blood.[31]

How to Avoid: Look for the label TB117-2013 on furniture, pillows, and other home goods, which indicates it doesn't contain chemical flame retardants. Otherwise, call the manufacturers to find out if chemical flame retardants were added. Look for furniture, car seats, and other products, made from wool or polyester, which are naturally flame-resistant. Dust, where flame retardants can accumulate, can account for up to 82 percent of our exposure, so remember to dust, vacuum, and mop frequently.[32] Don't reupholster older furniture or replace carpeting yourself.

Stain- and water-repellent treatments are found in the fabric used in furniture, carpets, clothing, shoes, and other goods. These treatments often contain perfluorochemicals like PFAS, which have been linked to cancer, thyroid dysfunction, immune system damage, liver issues, and a host of other health problems.[33] Making matters worse, PFAS-treated furniture doesn't even always repel water and stains more than untreated fabrics! According to research, the type of fabric and how you treat the stains matter more for repelling water and stains.[34] When I want water-repellent fabric, I opt for merino wool, which repels water naturally, and I use natural essential oils like lemon to help eliminate stains, which you can apply directly to most fabrics.

How to Avoid: Don't buy products marketed as stain- or water-repellent. To protect furniture, use a washable nonvinyl cover and vacuum regularly. Treat stains with castile soap, vinegar, hydrogen peroxide, and/or club soda—look online to see which products treat which stains most effectively. Some clothing manufacturers like Levi Strauss have already stopped using PFAS in their clothing, while other brands like Patagonia, L.L. Bean, Lululemon, and Eddie Bauer have promised to phase out the chemicals in coming years.[35] When in doubt, contact manufacturers to find out what's in your favorite brands.

Vinyl chloride/polyvinyl chloride (PVC) is found in patio furniture, windows, vinyl siding, flooring, children's and pet toys, shower curtains and liners, yoga mats, drinking-water pipes, and other plastic home goods. This known carcinogen can cause headaches, dizziness, and difficulty breathing, in addition to increasing the risk of miscarriage and birth defects among pregnant women.[36] The EPA is set to review whether to ban vinyl chloride—a flammable gas used to make PVC for plastic consumer goods—but the process could take several years.[37]

How to Avoid: Swap plastic patio furniture for sustainable teak or polyethylene wicker, and never buy plastic shower curtains or liners—use those made from tightly woven cotton, linen, or polyester instead. Research toys and yoga mats to make sure they don't contain PVC. If you are building or renovating your home, avoid PVC windows, pipes, vinyl siding, and flooring, opting for nontoxic materials instead.

Formaldehyde is found in pressed wood, particle board, and plywood furniture, cabinets, flooring, paneling, foam insulation, wallpaper, paint, and permanent-press clothing and curtains. As we've covered extensively, formaldehyde is a known carcinogen that's been linked to a host of other serious health problems.[38] Enough said.

How to Avoid: Don't buy pressed wood, particle board, or plywood furniture or cabinets. If you're tempted to purchase any of these products, look for items that specify they meet no-added-formaldehyde (NAF) requirements. When painting or repainting, opt for zero-VOC paint and forgo wallpaper. When building or remodeling, don't use foam insulation or pressed wood, particle board, or plywood in your paneling or flooring. Don't buy permanent-press or "wrinkle-free" bed linens, clothing, or curtains.

NOW THAT YOU know what VOCs are and how best to avoid them, I want to call attention to specific product categories so that the next time you're in the market for a new home item, you can consult this list. Alternatively, if you have the resources to replace items you already own, consider it preventative medicine and money well spent, with the ability to protect you and your family's health today, tomorrow, and beyond. Here's what to know about each product category:

Mattress and bedding. Most of us spend at least several hours per night in bed, which is why the type of mattress and bedding we use matters so much. Many commercial brands can emit VOCs from harmful chemicals like pesticides, flame retardants, PVC, and polyurethane foam. To avoid VOCs, shop for a mattress and bedding made from at least 95 percent Global Organic Textile Standard (GOTS)-certified organic cotton. If you can't afford organic, look for mattresses made from 100 percent natural latex or a low-VOC foam certified by an independent organization like OEKO-TEX or Greenguard. Avoid mattresses and bedding made with flame retardants, antimicrobials, or synthetic fragrances (none of which any certified organic cotton items can contain by law). Don't buy waterproof or PVC mattresses or pillow covers and opt instead for a tightly woven fabric like cotton or wool if you want to protect your bed or pillows.[39]

Furniture. Don't buy furniture imported from tropical countries, as it might have been sprayed with pesticides. Products manufactured in Europe, however, have to meet strict European Union standards for VOCs emissions. When shopping for American brands, look for furniture certified nontoxic by an independent organization; smart options include Greenguard, OEKO-TEX, GOTS, and Green Seal.[40] As we've covered, you'll want to choose furniture made without flame retardants (contact manufacturer if unsure) and avoid all stain- and water-resistant or waterproof products. Avoid plastic, plywood, particle board, and pressed wood furniture whenever possible.

Gas appliances. Gas stoves and other appliances, like washers and dryers, can emit a number of toxins, including carbon monoxide and benzene, a known carcinogen. When these appliances run their course in your home—or if you truly want to be proactive about your toxin exposure—replace them with electric appliances. In the meantime, improve your indoor air quality by always using a fan when you cook with gas, and open windows when you cook or do laundry.

OFF-GASSING 101

Almost all new products, including furniture, mattresses, bedding, carpets, clothing, flooring, paneling, and paint, can off-gas, or release VOCs and other chemicals into indoor air.[41] For this reason, don't stay or sleep in rooms that have recently been remodeled or painted without airing out the room first by opening windows and using fans for a sustained time. Similarly, every time you buy a new product or pick up your dry cleaning (see page 198), allow it time to off-gas on a covered deck or in your garage. While there's no definitive number of hours or days that will guarantee a safe product, off-gassing as often and as long as possible can help reduce indoor air pollution. Opening windows and ensuring proper ventilation can also help limit noxious gasses released from home products and building materials.

Electronics. You likely already know that computers, tablets, TVs, cell phones, and other electronic devices can emit sleep-disrupting blue light and contribute to mood disorders by providing endless access to anxiety-inducing email, doom-scrolling news sources, and comparison-invoking social media. But there's another way these products interfere with our health: many contain phthalates, lead, brominated flame retardants, and PVC. That's why these products, along with their cords and cables, have to be recycled carefully. While the chemicals in electronics can be difficult to avoid, you can limit your exposure by washing your hands after use and dusting frequently.

Another concern with electronics and the wireless technology on which they rely is low-level electric and magnetic fields (EMF) radiation, which can alter human cells and possibly increase the risk of cancer, fertility problems, development issues in children, and unfavorable birth outcomes in unborn children.[42] To reduce your exposure to EMF radiation, keep computers, phones, and other devices away from your body as often as possible, particularly away from your head and reproductive organs. Don't rest your laptop on your groin or keep your smartphone near your breasts. Use headphones or a speakerphone when making calls whenever possible or simply text. Don't carry your phone in your pants pocket or bra; radiation absorption decreases substantially with even a little bit of separation. That's why I always tell patients that distance is your friend when it comes to EMF radiation exposure.

If you keep your phone near your bed at night, switch it onto airplane mode while you sleep to reduce radiation. If you're pregnant, keep phones and computers away from your belly, and if you already have children, limit their time on the devices or download games to your phone or tablet, then switch to airplane mode while they play. Finally, don't use a "radiation shield" for your cell phone, as the gimmick can cause devices to paradoxically emit more radiation in the effort to connect.[43]

Carpets. Chemicals in conventional carpeting can contribute significantly to indoor air pollution. For this reason, the EWG recommends avoiding wall-to-wall carpeting and swapping out conventional carpets for solid wood flooring, tile, cork, or natural linoleum (with a low-VOC finish or sealant) whenever possible. If you do want a carpet, choose one made from wool with a wool or felt backing instead of those made from synthetic fabric and that have a synthetic rubber or PVC backing. For area rugs, look for wool or natural fibers like jute, seagrass, or sisal. If you do go synthetic, be sure to get a seal from Greenguard or Green Label Plus for both the carpet and the padding, which indicate lower VOC emissions. Avoid stain and water-resistant treatments, and when installing new carpet, vent well to reduce exposure to flame retardants in the old carpeting. Finally, consider adopting a "no-shoes" policy to limit your tracking in harmful pollutants and vacuum frequently, using only water if you steam-clean.[44]

Clothing. The textile industry uses fabrics that are immensely toxic, with many containing a ton of chemicals like PFAS, BPA, lead, chromium, phthalates, bleach, and synthetic dyes.[45] This is true of intimate clothing like underwear and even what we use to exercise in, and sweating can increase chemical absorption because the skin pores are more open and absorbent. This is especially troubling given a recent study from the Center for Environmental Health that found many major brands of activewear expose people to up to forty times the safe limit for BPA.[46]

To reduce your risk, remove activewear immediately after exercise and shower soon after to remove chemical residue. Choose loose-fitting certified organic cotton for activities that don't require tightly fitted material. For day-to-day wear, opt for clothing made from certified organic cotton or 100 percent wool or silk. When buying synthetic, look for clothing with third-party certification from OEKO-TEX Standard

100, GOTS, and EU Ecolabel.[47] Avoid stain- and water-resistant shoes and apparel, along with permanent press and wrinkle-free, as both emit high levels of VOCs.

Pet supplies. Flea and tick medicine and conventional cat litter, especially if it contains fragrance, can be toxic to you and your pets. Replace flea and tick collars and sprays with those made from essential oils only, and use an all-natural material like sawdust for litter boxes. If you must use conventional litter, opt for non-scented varieties and wear a mask when handling.

DEADLY DRY CLEANING: THE DIRTY TRUTH ABOUT THE POPULAR CLEANING SERVICE

It can feel especially fancy to pick up a piece of clothing from the dry cleaners, the service somehow transforming our most wrinkled or stained shirts, skirts, dresses, or pants into pieces that appear brand new again. But dry cleaning—which isn't actually dry but, rather, involves the use of many "wet" chemicals—is one of the most toxic services to which we can subscribe, thanks in part to a particularly noxious compound known as perchloroethylene (PERC), used by most conventional cleaners. Not only is PERC listed as a probable carcinogen by the International Agency for Research on Cancer, but it can also interfere with nervous system function and cause liver and kidney damage, impaired memory, reproductive harm, and other serious health effects.[48] Another problem with PERC is that it doesn't leave our bodies easily; it can accumulate in our fat cells over time.[49]

The overall health ramifications of dry cleaning are so serious that if you live in an area with a high density of dry cleaners, you may have up to a 27 percent greater chance of developing kidney cancer, according to one study that examined hospital discharge rates in New York City over a ten-year period. Those researchers discovered that people diagnosed with kidney cancer were more likely to hail from zip codes in New York with a high density of PERC-using drying cleaners[50]—one reason why the city now offers free chemical testing for those living in apartments above or adjacent to dry-cleaning shops.[51] Chemicals like PERC are also strongly implicated in the development of scleroderma, an autoimmune disease that can cause the hardening or tightening of skin, leading to potential digestive troubles, heart and lung problems, and other health issues.

Even if the nearest dry cleaners is miles from you, if you regularly get clothes dry cleaned, you are being exposed to PERC. In fact, people who bring dry-cleaned clothing inside their homes have two- to sixfold higher levels of PERC in their bodies than those who aren't directly exposed to dry cleaning, according to research.[52]

Studies also show that dry-cleaned clothing can release PERC for up to forty-eight hours afterward, which is why leaving items outside your home to off-gas on a covered deck or in a garage is critical. Then, after at least two days of off-gassing, wear undershirts, tank tops, or slips under chemically cleaned clothing to limit your skin absorption.

It's important to note, however, that these precautions won't obviate your exposure to PERC, so instead of using dry cleaning, consider an old-fashioned iron or steam cleaner to remove wrinkles at home. If you do choose to dry-clean, look for less toxic alternatives that spot-clean, steam, or hand-wash with mild detergents or liquid carbon dioxide, which is a "truly green dry-cleaning method," according to the EPA.

The household cleaners you use, the type of furniture and other home goods you buy, and even your clothing and how you clean it can all contribute to indoor air pollution. Thankfully, cleaning up your indoor air doesn't mean throwing out everything you own; rather, you can make smarter, safer choices whenever you purchase new items and learn how to clean in a simple way that can save you money while increasing the sparkle of your home and your family's health.

Chapter 7 Takeaways

- Use the EWG's Guide to Healthy Cleaning to buy safe and effective all-natural cleaners or make your own cleaning solutions. The latter are totally safe, just as effective, and oftentimes much more economical (see recipes in Appendix 3).
- Keep all new furniture, bedding, and any other purchases in a garage or protected outside area for several days to allow them to "off-gas" chemicals.
- Whenever you buy a new item for your home, choose a cleaner alternative using the suggestions outlined in this chapter and looking for third-party seal or certifications, like those from Greenguard, OEKO-TEX Standard 100, GOTS, or EU Ecolabel.
- Dust daily or every other day whenever possible, and invest in a vacuum with a HEPA filter: Dust can collect harmful volatile organic compounds (VOCs) and be a major source of indoor air pollution.
- Choose 100 percent organic cotton, silk, and wool clothing whenever possible, and follow smart safety steps when wearing exercise apparel.
- Since conventional dry cleaning can be toxic, iron or steam-clean clothing at home or look for less toxic commercial alternatives that use liquid carbon dioxide or water and mild detergents to clean.

SECTION III

ADD

CHAPTER 8
Using Food to Detoxify

NO MATTER HOW vigilant you are about avoiding toxins in your everyday life, no one can avoid all chemical exposure all the time. That's true of every one of us, no matter where we choose to live or travel, what we do for a living, or how mindful we are of our behavior. While the twenty-first century has seen some incredible developments that have improved many aspects of our daily lives, one downside to modern-day living is our surplus of modern-day chemicals, many of them highly toxic to human health.

Science may have created the chemical industry, but it has also shown us that we possess a powerful advantage against today's toxins that's as old as humankind itself: our body's natural, built-in ability to detoxify. Thanks to modern-day research, we know that our body is really good at getting rid of chemicals. It's an evolutionary adaptation dating back to when our ancient ancestors were exposed to natural chemicals in the water, food, woodsmoke, and other sources. We also know that there are specific, science-backed ways to improve the body's ability to detoxify, which in turn can help reduce the impact of those environmental exposures we simply can't avoid.

When it comes to detoxification, though, science is key. While some may claim certain supplements, foods, or therapies help "clean" the body, many of these claims aren't substantiated by valid studies—and some claims, like doing colonics, undertaking restrictive juice cleanses, or buying specific supplements, may do more harm than good. That's why you'll read only about the lifestyle changes that work in this chapter and the following one, along with the research to show that they can and do help the body better eliminate environmental toxins.

I'm living proof that you can improve your body's ability to detoxify with minor lifestyle changes. Some of the most effective detoxifying habits, which are covered in the next chapter, include boosting how long or how often you exercise or sweat, improving how long or what kind of sleep you get, and adopting active ways to manage stress, even if you don't believe you're acutely stressed. In this chapter, however, I focus on the two most effective ways to increase your body's natural detoxification processes:

- Consuming specific foods and supplements that have been shown to speed the rate and efficacy at which your body can eliminate toxins.
- Working to build what I call "nutritional sufficiency," when the body has the nutrients it needs to function fully and can leverage its built-in detox pathways, including the liver, kidneys, lungs, skin, and other major organs and systems.

My Detoxification Story

Most Americans lack nutritional sufficiency, even those who eat healthy, because we're constantly exposed to toxins (and medications) that interfere with optimal nutritional absorption. Also, food today is less nutritious owing to reduced soil quality compared to decades ago. A national survey of more than sixteen thousand Americans also found that we don't eat as nutritionally as we think we do, with 94 percent of people not consuming adequate amounts of vitamin E through diet, and 52 percent and 44 percent don't get enough magnesium and calcium, respectively.[1] Vitamin D is another pervasive nutrient deficiency, with 1 billion people around the globe estimated to be deficient.[2] But without adequate nutritional sufficiency, we can't take full advantage of our body's ability to detoxify.

More than fifteen years ago, shortly after my husband and I bought our dream house on two hundred acres of farmland in central New Jersey, we learned that the people who owned the farmland adjacent to us—essentially our backyard—were spraying it liberally with glyphosate, the active ingredient in Roundup and the most widely used herbicide in the United States, which research has shown may increase cancer risk by more than 40 percent.[3] While my husband and I already knew farmers had amply used pesticides on the land for years, this revelation caused my internal alert system to go ballistic. In lieu of moving, I knew we had to do everything we could to help our bodies better get rid of toxins, particularly glyphosate.

Before we did anything, though, I had both my husband and I get urine tests for glyphosate so that we knew what our exposure was at the time. The analysis, while not common back then, was still relatively easy and inexpensive to do. (Today, it's even easier and less expensive; see page 297 to learn more on blood testing for glyphosate.) The reason I felt it was important for us to test before doing anything was that, as an evidence-based doctor, I try to rely on available data before acting, so that I'm making the most informed decisions about my health and the health of my patients and family. In the case of glyphosate, I wanted a barometer to gauge if and by how much our exposure was affecting our bodies, and if and by how much we could lower that exposure over time.

When we got our test results back, I was alarmed but not surprised to learn that we both had troubling glyphosate levels. But I didn't want to let our numbers scare me. As an evidence-based doctor, I also believe in being proactive, rather than reactive, about my health. Now was the time to act, and the best way to act, as I was learning, was to double down on reducing the points of chemical exposures I could control. So I started eating more organic foods, being extra-vigilant about my drinking water, and following all the action steps discussed so far in this book. At the same time, I began using food to help remove pesticides and other toxins from my body, aiming to reduce the points of exposure I couldn't control.

My husband and I had always eaten relatively healthy, but after I saw our glyphosate numbers, I knew healthy wasn't enough. While eating healthy is both incredible and incredibly commendable, it's not necessarily a guarantee you're consuming the specific healthy foods shown to boost the body's ability to detoxify. What's more, even if you follow a healthy diet, you still may not have *nutritional sufficiency*, which occurs when the body has adequate levels of all the nutrients it needs to function optimally, maximizing its ability to detoxify. If you don't have nutritional sufficiency, your body can't efficiently combat inflammation or optimize its top detoxifying pathways: the liver, the kidneys, the skin, and the respiratory, circulatory, and lymphatic systems.

What are the most detoxifying foods you can consume, and how do you achieve nutritional sufficiency? That's what this chapter is all about, but first, let's go back to my glyphosate story.

AT THE TIME my husband and I had our levels tested, I was studying integrative medicine with Dr. Andrew Weil at the Center for Integrative Medicine at the University of Arizona. While I already had my medical degree in internal medicine and was a practicing rheumatologist, I wanted to better understand how to prevent and treat disease at the core—what integrative medicine is all about. Compared to conventional medicine, which primarily teaches doctors (even today) to ameliorate health issues with prescription drugs and invasive procedures, I wanted to treat medical problems upstream at their source.

During my work with Dr. Andrew Weil, who is an international thought leader in both integrative medicine and preventative nutrition, I discovered how critical certain foods can be to boosting the body's ability to eliminate toxins. Near the top of the list are cruciferous vegetables, a category that includes hundreds of veggies like broccoli, cabbage, bok choy, and collard greens, all which contain specific compounds shown to promote liver detoxification.[4] I have a family history of breast cancer, and I was aware that consuming higher quantities of these special veggies could prolong remission in women with the disease; in fact, scientists are developing a cancer drug made from cruciferous-veggie compounds.[5] After learning about their specific detoxifying properties back then, though, I was ready to get on board with a whole lot more than bok choy.

So, my husband and I began eating cruciferous vegetables every day, making sure we got at least one large serving of the veggies daily. Before you think "boring," "snooze," or "OMG, how can I do that with work and kids?" know that consuming more cruciferous veggies was a fun and relatively easy culinary adventure. Because there are so many cruciferous veggies (see page 215 for a full list) we made it our mission to try a new one every month.

This is how we learned, for example, that raw kohlrabi is delicious as a cracker substitute for hummus and other dips, and that Chinese daikon radish is a great way to add color and crunch to salads. These days, there are even more innovative ways to add cruciferous veggies to your diet, given the popularity of recipes that substitute cauliflower, turnip, rutabaga, and other veggies from the group for flour, potatoes, rice, and other carb-heavy foods. (See Appendix 4 for my delicious detox recipes, including Apple Bok Choy Salad and Cauliflower Risotto.)

After my husband and I got into an everyday routine of eating (and enjoying) more cruciferous veggies, I suggested we start targeting foods known to increase *glutathione*, a vital antioxidant shown to remove chemicals like mercury, arsenic, dioxins, and herbicides like glyphosate from the body.[6] While I'll talk much more about glutathione in the next few pages, I can't emphasize enough how critical it is to good health—so much so that functional medicine expert Dr. Mark Hyman calls it both "the most important molecule you need to stay healthy and prevent disease" and "the mother of all antioxidants, the master detoxifier, and the maestro of the immune system."[7]

Some foods contain glutathione while others, like asparagus, spinach, avocado, green beans, and papaya,[8] increase the body's ability to manufacture the powerful antioxidant, made by the liver. Foods high in sulfur (like cruciferous veggies), selenium, and the B vitamins also help the body manufacture the antioxidant. Finally, foods like nuts, seeds, and lentils all contain the amino acid cysteine, one of the three building blocks that make up glutathione. (Animal meat, seafood, and dairy products like yogurt also contain cysteine; just be sure to choose organic versions when possible, for all the reasons discussed in previous chapters). When I learned about how critical glutathione is for detoxification, my husband and I started consuming more of all these foods.

The more I worked with Dr. Weil, the more adamant I became about shaping our diet around detoxifying foods. At the same time, though, I knew whatever we ate to detoxify wouldn't be as effective if we didn't have nutritional sufficiency. While many nutrients are needed for complete nutritional sufficiency, I began by targeting those that we often don't get enough of: the B vitamins, vitamin D_3, and the two types of marine omega-3s—docosahexaenoic acid (DHA) and eicosapentaenoic acid (EPA).

I also started eating more probiotic-rich foods after learning how a healthy microbiome helps the body better eliminate toxins while preventing chemicals from entering the bloodstream. (This is the basis for the concept of leaky gut syndrome that we talked about on page 41.) The trillions of healthy microorganisms that live in your gut microbiome can break down harmful chemicals in the gut; for example, various strains of the healthy bacteria *Lactobacillus*, found in some fermented foods like yogurt, can bind to lead and other heavy metals in the gut, helping the body better eliminate them. What's more, having more healthy microbes bolsters the strength of your intestinal lining, preventing leaky gut, protecting toxins from entering the bloodstream, and helping the body better move chemicals down and out your gastrointestinal tract.

I began to make sure I had at least one serving of probiotics every day, whether it was organic yogurt, sauerkraut, or salt-brined, fermented pickles (which contain more healthy bacteria than those brined in vinegar). I also increased my intake of vinegar, which bolsters gut health, by adding balsamic vinegar to salads or creating my own dressing from apple cider vinegar mixed with honey. Finally, I began taking a high-quality probiotic supplement—one of the four fundamental supplements I recommend everyone take daily—because modern life can make it difficult for any of us to build up enough healthy bacteria (as you'll read about on page 247).

We also got into contact with the farmers who owned the land behind our home, asking them to alert us when they were spraying their fields with glyphosate so that we could close all our windows and doors, leave our home for the day, and board our pets or at least be sure to keep them inside. Remember: you have a say in your own health, and personal advocacy, in whatever form you give it, has a place in protecting your body from environmental toxins.

During this time of expanding my detoxification pathways, I began to view the body as a human filtration system. I realized that the more water we drank, and the faster and more efficiently our body could move that water through our liver and kidneys, the faster and more effectively our body would filter out toxins. As humans, we're similar to the lakes in which we like to swim and fish: the more water a lake has, and the more frequently it moves that water through its natural filtration system (like rocks, soil, and sediment), the less polluted the lake will be. Otherwise, a lake without a continual source of new water or adequate water movement will become stagnant.

For these reasons, I started drinking forty to sixty ounces of water in the course of the day—the equivalent of two to three standard twenty-ounce water bottles—while also preparing foods with herbs like dandelion greens, which act as a strong natural diuretic. (Before adding any diuretic foods or supplements to your diet, always consult your healthcare practitioner, especially if you have a medical condition that may be affected by a change in your daily water intake, like a kidney issue or high blood pressure.) My goal was balance, as foods like dandelion greens, when consumed alongside plenty of water, can help the body more quickly flush out excess salts, fluids, and toxins.

If this sounds like I became obsessed with countering our glyphosate exposure, you're right. But I viewed our situation the same way as someone who works for OSHA (Occupational Safety and Health Administration) might look at an employee who handles toxins every day as part of their job: My husband and I were exposed to high doses of the same chemical for hours on end, every day, which was similar to someone who has an occupational chemical hazard. And while we didn't test our two young sons, we implemented the same dietary changes with them, as I knew they were in an even more vulnerable period for exposure (see pages 54–61 for vulnerable periods of exposure). They may have grumbled about all the broccoli and other cruciferous vegetables, and were resistant to dandelion greens at first, but kids develop tastes young, and introducing them to new foods, especially when prepared in simple, tasty ways, can set their diet for a lifetime. Heck, lots of kids learn to love spinach, so why not do the same thing with dandelion greens?

Whether obsessive or not, my hypervigilance paid off. Two years after my husband and I first tested for glyphosate, the concentration of the chemical in our urine had dropped to a level below normal. We accomplished that without changing our exposure to the toxin; we continued to live next to two hundred acres of farmland that was sprayed just as frequently with glyphosate as it had been when we first moved into our home. What did change, though, was our diet.

Fifteen years later, I still prioritize detoxifying foods each day while taking my "human fertilizer" supplements, including a high-quality multivitamin (which you'll learn about in just a moment). I believe these supplements are necessary to provide the nutritional sufficiency that helps the body thrive. I've also learned how to cook easy, detoxifying meals with foods that have the nutrients shown to help the body both protect itself from and better eliminate environmental toxins. (You'll find my favorite recipes in Appendix 4.)

None of this is to say that changing your diet alone is all you need to do to fight environmental exposure. Because we're barraged with countless toxins every day in our water, food, personal-care products, and indoor and outdoor atmosphere, we need to do everything possible to reduce those points of exposure if we want to be healthy and prevent the potential onset of environmentally related symptoms and disease. And while a detoxifying diet *may* treat or reverse symptoms or illnesses caused by environmental exposure, it's not a guarantee, by any means. Still, whether you're concerned about a specific chemical or you simply want to do everything you can to be as healthy as possible, prioritizing a detoxifying diet is one of the best ways to do that. You'll be supporting your detoxifying pathways to increase your body's ability to eliminate harmful chemicals.

In this chapter, we start by looking at the top eight foods or food groups you can consume to help your body better detoxify. Then, I detail my four "human fertilizer" supplements that I believe everyone should take for nutritional sufficiency, no matter your diet. (Note: Always consult a healthcare practitioner before taking any supplements.)

My Top Eight Detoxifying Foods

Cruciferous vegetables. These vegetables, a group that includes more than three thousand species, are loaded with glucosinolates, the amazing sulfur-rich compounds that increase the liver's production of detoxifying enzymes, in addition to helping curb inflammation and preventing and slowing cancer growth, according to the research.[9] When you eat lots of cruciferous veggies, especially broccoli and broccoli sprouts, you'll up your intake of sulforaphane, a by-product of glucosinolate shown to induce the liver to undertake its most effective detoxifying phase, known as the *conjugation*, when toxins are neutralized and excreted.[10] Studies also show that sulforaphane increases glutathione, the body's "master" antioxidant that improves liver detoxification and protects cells from inflammation.[11]

Cruciferous veggies also contain compounds that regulate natural estrogen metabolism. This is key to preventing and treating hormone-dependent cancers, while negating certain harmful effects of endocrine-disrupting chemicals (EDCs). What's more, these veggies are packed with fiber—one cup of chopped broccoli (cooked or raw) contains 5 grams of fiber—which can speed toxin elimination by increasing how quickly the body excretes chemicals and other waste products. Cruciferous veggies also contain prebiotic fibers that feed the healthy gut microbes, helping increase the number of good bacteria in the microbiome.[12] Healthy gut microbes are important for detoxification, since good bacteria can neutralize certain toxins while working to fortify the intestinal lining to prevent chemicals from entering the bloodstream.

As you know from my own story, when it comes to cruciferous veggies you're not limited to broccoli, Brussels sprouts, and cauliflower. There are literally hundreds of different types to try, including those in the list that follows, so experiment to find what you like. I recommend eating a total of two to five cups daily of any of these for optimal benefits. Many recipes in Appendix 4 are for cruciferous veggies, and some of my favorites include Broccoli Slaw (page 311) and Apple Bok Choy Salad (page 312)!

- Arugula
- Bok choy
- Broccoli ✓
- Broccoli rabe ✓
- Broccoli romanesco
- Brussels sprouts ✓
- Cabbage ✓
- Cauliflower ✓
- Chinese broccoli
- Chinese cabbage
- Collard greens
- Daikon radish
- Garden cress
- Horseradish
- Kale
- Kohlrabi
- Mizuna
- Mustard greens
- Radish
- Rutabaga
- Turnips ✓
- Wasabi
- Watercress

PRO TIP: HOW TO COOK BROCCOLI TO INCREASE ITS DETOXIFYING ABILITY

To boost the detoxifying benefits of broccoli, trim and chop the veggie into small pieces first, then allow the pieces to sit for at least forty minutes before cooking. Studies have found that cutting up broccoli and other cruciferous veggies and then exposing the pieces to air helps activate an enzyme called myrosinase, which helps turn glucosinolate into sulforaphane. Because some forms of cooking can reduce sulforaphane, the higher the quantity of the nutrient in the veggie before cooking, the more you'll increase your total intake of it.[13] Raw cruciferous veggies, like broccoli, contain the most sulforaphane, and prepping them using this method can help retain the compound even after cooking, preferably by stir-frying or by sous vide briefly.

Alliums. This class of flowering plants, which includes onions, garlic, scallions, shallots, leeks, and chives, is packed with sulfur-rich molecules known as *organosulfur compounds*, which help give these veggies their strong odor and flavor. Like sulforaphane, organosulfur compounds stimulate the liver to break down toxins, then neutralize them during the organ's more effective conjugation phase.[14] Similar to cruciferous veggies, alliums have been studied for their potential to fight cancer, with studies showing they may interfere with cancer-cell growth.[15] Onions are also one of the best dietary sources of quercetin, an antioxidant shown to reduce cancer risk and protect the body from certain chemicals like mercury and polychlorinated biphenyls (PCBs; see page 219 for more on this).[16] And all alliums, which are rich in sulfur, have been shown to increase glutathione, the body's "master" detoxifying antioxidant.[17] Aim to eat alliums daily, and for increased health benefits, mix them with extra-virgin olive oil, which makes the healthy compounds more usable by the body for anti-inflammatory health benefits. Crush garlic cloves before sautéing or roasting to increase their detoxifying nutrients.[18] Aim to eat as much of these as possible, as there's no risk to your health—only more fiber and other healthy nutrients to enjoy. I often sauté sweet onions or shallots in extra-virgin olive oil and sea salt to soften them and make them sweeter before adding them to other dishes.

Many recipes in Appendix 4 use alliums, but some of my favorites include Curried Cauliflower (page 316), Cauliflower Risotto (page 315), Paleo Grass-Fed Beef or Lamb Hash (page 320), and Carrot Ginger Soup (page 310).

Foods that increase glutathione production. Research shows that this antioxidant compound, found in many foods and also made by the body, can break down both endogenous and exogenous toxins, including environmental chemicals.[19] Glutathione, which is made up of three amino acids—cysteine, glycine, and glutamic acid—also neutralizes damaging inflammatory substances known as free radicals and may help transport mercury out of the cells. Chronic exposure to environmental toxins and drinking too much alcohol have been shown to deplete glutathione, increasing the risk of premature aging and chronic conditions like autoimmune disease, Alzheimer's, and liver disease.[20]

Some foods contain glutathione: avocado, asparagus, green beans, cucumber, papaya, and spinach are among the best plant sources. But it's unclear if we can properly absorb the antioxidant from foods. Other foods have high levels of cysteine, one of glutathione's three amino acids. Good sources of cysteine include cow's dairy, chicken and pork, wheat germ, lentils, oatmeal, eggs, and sunflower seeds.

As mentioned, sulfur-rich foods like cruciferous veggies and alliums can also increase glutathione levels. Chop or crush the vegetables to activate the bioactive molecules that increase glutathione enzyme activity, and stick to steaming or eating them raw for maximum benefits. Green tea, grape juice, rosemary, milk thistle, and the spice turmeric have all been shown to do the same.[21]

Unfortunately, no matter how many glutathione-boosting foods you consume, you may not be able to increase your antioxidant levels if you don't have nutritional sufficiency. That's because your body needs many nutrients to make glutathione, including B vitamins, vitamins C and E, omega-3 fatty acids, and selenium, among others.[22] This is one reason I recommend my patients take a daily omega-3 supplement, along with a multivitamin that has B vitamins, vitamins C and E, and selenium (as explained on page 231). Finally, lifestyle plays an important role in glutathione production, so be sure to prioritize getting enough high-quality sleep and exercise, both of which help detoxify the body in other ways.

Many recipes in Appendix 4 contain glutathione or nutrients that boost the production of the antioxidant, but some of my favorites include Creamy Cauliflower Soup (page 307), Broccoli Slaw (page 311), Carrot Ginger Soup (page 310), Lemony Brussels Sprouts Slaw (page 313), Blueberry Chia Seed Pudding (page 323), and Avocado and Berry Ice Cream (page 325).

Foods that contain quercetin. Quercetin is an antioxidant and flavonoid, a class of plant chemicals found in vegetables, fruits, dark chocolate, and wine, shown to have anticancer and anti-inflammatory properties. According to research, quercetin in particular helps increase glutathione production and prevents oxidative stress, which occurs when there's an imbalance of free radicals and antioxidants in the body.[23] When it comes to detoxifying from environmental chemicals, the research on quercetin is impressive, with studies showing it helps chelate (extract from the body) heavy metals like lead, cadmium, and mercury. Scientists also call quercetin "one of the most impressive drugs" to mitigate detrimental effects to the heart caused by pesticide exposure.[24] Additionally, the antioxidant may reduce liver damage from polychlorinated bisphenols (PCBs), according to animal studies.[25] I suggest patients with asthma, allergies, hives, or other allergic reactions consume more quercetin-containing foods, as the antioxidant has also been shown to curb histamine, a chemical released by the immune system and responsible in part for triggering allergic responses.[26]

To eat more quercetin, choose red onions, one of the best dietary sources of the nutrient, followed by white onions, red-leaf lettuce, capers, apples, hot green chiles, black plums, cranberries, herbs like cilantro and dill, and a handful of other plant-based foods. If you want to take a quercetin supplement, I recommend 400 to 600 milligrams taken three times daily on an empty stomach along with vitamin C, which helps optimize absorption. As always, speak with your doctor before taking any supplement.

For recipes in Appendix 4 that include quercetin-promoting ingredients, check out Quick Gazpacho (page 310), Apple Bok Choy Salad (page 312), and Lemony Brussels Sprouts Slaw (page 313).

Foods that contain selenium. This essential mineral ("essential" means we need it to survive) plays a critical role in the body, helping regulate thyroid hormones, protect cells from oxidative stress, and repair DNA damage.[27] While all these functions aid in detoxification, selenium is a real star at helping eliminate environmental chemicals, as shown by studies, and counteracting toxicity from heavy metals like mercury and cadmium.[28] One study out of Japan even found that people who consume a lot of whale meat, which is high in mercury yet also has high selenium levels, didn't suffer adverse effects from the mercury exposure.[29] Several animal studies have also found that selenium may protect the body from bisphenol A (BPA)[30] and mitigate the harmful effects of air pollution.[31] Finally, as a rheumatologist, I'm impressed by research showing that the trace mineral may reduce complications from autoimmune conditions and improve survival rates.[32]

Many foods contain selenium, but Brazil nuts are the best source: A single one of these nuts contains more than what you need per day, with 68 to 91 micrograms of the mineral per nut, slightly above the recommended daily allowance (RDA) of 55 micrograms for men and women. Seafood like tuna, sardines, and halibut is also a rich source of selenium, and it's also found in lower levels in beef, pork, poultry, rice, eggs, oatmeal, and dairy. With selenium, though, more is not better:

too much of the mineral can cause toxicity. This is why you shouldn't consume more than two Brazil nuts per day or take selenium as a standalone supplement if you already have a multivitamin with the mineral. Symptoms of overconsuming selenium include hair loss, fatigue, muscle tenderness, gastrointestinal symptoms, and neurological problems.[33]

For recipes in Appendix 4 that are high in selenium, see Creamy Cauliflower Soup (page 307), Pureed Butternut Squash Soup (page 308), Barley Miso Soup (page 309), Breakfast Challenge Turkey Chili (page 319), Asparagus in Balsamic Butter (page 318), and Ginger Lemon Truffles (page 324).

Foods that contain turmeric. If you've ever had South Asian or Middle Eastern food, you've likely tasted turmeric, a pungent, bright orange spice made from the root of *Curcuma longa*, a flowering plant native to Southeast Asia. Turmeric is found in curry powder and some mustards, and is used on its own to flavor many classic Moroccan, Thai, Vietnamese, Indian, and Indonesian dishes. Not only flavorful, turmeric is also incredibly healthy, thanks to the active compound curcumin. Research shows that curcumin is a powerful antioxidant and anti-inflammatory, and it can help prevent conditions related to chronic systemic inflammation, like cancer, heart disease, Alzheimer's, Parkinson's, diabetes, obesity, arthritis, and depression.[34]

When it comes to detoxification, research shows that curcumin helps counter oxidative stress, neutralize free radicals, and increase enzymes that assist the body in metabolizing toxins.[35] The compound may also counteract the effects of mercury toxicity[36] and protect brain cells from the damaging effects of lead and cadmium, according to animal studies.[37] Curcumin may also increase glutathione, boosting its anti-inflammatory and anticancer effects, per research.[38]

To consume more turmeric (and curcumin, as a result), use the spice liberally, adding 1 to 4 teaspoons of a USDA organic product to increase flavor and provide a deep yellow color to eggs, tofu, roasted vegetables, salad dressing, or smoothies. You can also try making tea from ground turmeric, lemon, and honey; if you add milk, you'll have the popular Indian drink known as golden milk tea. For ideal absorption, season your food or tea with a moderate amount of black pepper, which contains piperine, shown to increase the bioavailability of curcumin by 2,000 percent.[39] Otherwise, you may want to consider supplementing with curcumin; see page 233 for details.

For recipes in Appendix 4 that use turmeric, see Curried Cauliflower (page 316), Golden Milk (page 327), and Green Detox Smoothie (page 327).

Artichokes. This popular Mediterranean vegetable is a great way to boost liver health and function, both which can help increase the body's ability to detoxify. According to research, extracts from artichoke leaves and roots help protect the liver and can even trigger the regeneration of liver cells.[40] Artichoke extract has been found to significantly increase bile production for several hours, helping speed liver detoxification and lower blood cholesterol.[41] The vegetable has also been shown in animal studies to decrease liver inflammation and prevent liver disease.[42]

Aim to add five or more artichokes to your diet per week by steaming, roasting, grilling, pan-frying, microwaving, poaching, or stuffing them. Or include chopped artichoke hearts in salads, pizza, pastas, sauces, sandwiches, and dips. For recipes in Appendix 4 that use artichokes, see Cauliflower Risotto (page 315), Pulled Chicken, Squash, and Greens (page 321), Paleo Grass-Fed Beef or Lamb Hash (page 320), Breakfast Challenge Turkey Chili (page 319), and Moroccan-Style Chicken Stew (page 318).

Dandelions. This weed with a bright-yellow flower is an edible herb, one of the most detoxifying foods you can consume. The plant is rich in antioxidants, helping to counter the oxidative damage caused by environmental toxins. Dandelion has been used for centuries as a liver tonic, but research now exists to support the belief that dandelion helps protect and support liver function.[43] The herb is also a strong natural diuretic, helping the body move water and waste quickly and effectively from the cells. Compounds in dandelion may also fight chronic inflammation and lower blood sugar and cholesterol.[44]

I tell my patients to try to consume dandelions at least three times a week by stir-frying the plant's greens or adding them fresh to salads, or using the flowers to make tea. You can also buy dandelion tea or powdered dandelion root, which makes a delicious coffee substitute. Otherwise, look for fresh dandelion greens at your local farmers' market or supermarket, or harvest your own—just be sure they have not been sprayed with pesticides or other chemicals. You can also take dandelion in supplement form: talk with your practitioner before doing so and follow the label for dosing instructions.

For recipes in Appendix 4 that use dandelion, see Dandelion, Jícama, and Orange Prebiotic Salad (page 313) and Paleo Bok Choy Salad (page 314).

USE INTERMITTENT FASTING TO RAMP UP YOUR BODY'S ABILITY TO DETOXIFY

Intermittent fasting, which is eating at specific times and forgoing food during the remaining hours, has become a popular, science-backed way to lose weight, boost cognitive function, improve metabolism, reduce disease risk, and even slow the aging process.[45] While the strategy may be a trend today, the idea behind intermittent fasting is not new. Humans have restricted their caloric intake for millennia, or whenever food hasn't been readily available. More and more research has been showing that occasional caloric restriction helps protect the cells from environmental toxins and even purge chemicals from the body.[46]

One reason intermittent fasting acts as a detoxification boon is that prolonged calorie restriction tricks the body into believing it's in survival mode, triggering a process known as *autophagy*.[47] Autophagy is the body's equivalent of taking out its cellular trash, "cleaning" our tissues by removing inflammatory compounds and toxic waste products. Research also shows that intermittent fasting lowers inflammation in the immune system (oxidative stress), activates the production of detoxifying enzymes, and prompts the liver to increase its activity of liver detoxification.[48]

I intermittent-fast nearly every day, eating my first meal at noon and finishing with an early dinner at 5 p.m. It took me months to adapt to the schedule, and I break the pattern for special occasions or when I have a social evening out with friends or colleagues that mandates a later dinner. (This is a great example of the "allow" mindset, in which you allow adaptations and changes to your life based on what's happening in real time.) For most people, I recommend starting with a twelve-hour fast and twelve-hour feeding window, then increasing the fasting time over a period to last for sixteen to eighteen hours, with an eight- or six-hour feeding window, respectively.

To help get you through your fasting hours, drink as much unsweetened tea or coffee as you want, and make sure your first meal of the day after fasting, no matter when you choose to eat it, contains a good deal of protein and fiber, with a healthy fat like extra-virgin olive oil or nut butter to help stabilize blood sugar, which reduces hunger. Just be sure to consult with a practitioner before beginning a fasting program, especially if you have a metabolic health condition like diabetes.

Nutritional Sufficiency and My Four "Human Fertilizer" Supplements

In the beginning of this chapter, I shared my story about how I used food to improve my body's ability to detoxify. But I didn't do it with food alone: I also took several specific, high-quality dietary supplements. Why? Even though I had followed a healthy way of eating for years, I was concerned about my *nutritional sufficiency*—that optimal state when the body has adequate amounts of the nutrients it needs to function at full throttle. When we have nutritional sufficiency, our body has an easier time preventing epigenomic changes (or genetic changes that occur within our lifetime owing to diet and environment—see page 62 for more on this). Nutritional sufficiency also helps us produce glutathione and the other detoxifying enzymes and operate all our detoxifying organs, like the liver, kidneys, lungs, and skin, at 100 percent capacity.

While you can achieve nutritional sufficiency with food alone, it's difficult, for several reasons. For starters, food today isn't as nutritious as it used to be before the 1950s, due to industrial processing, soil depletion, and transport time from field or farm to kitchen table, all factors that can degrade nutrients. At the same time, we're exposed to more and more environmental toxins, which can deplete or interfere with our nutrient absorption. What's more, many common over-the-counter and prescription drugs can interfere with nutrient absorption, including the proton pump inhibitors used for acid reflux, which reduce calcium and B_{12} levels; and contraceptive pills, which can increase urinary excretion of a host of B vitamins in addition to vitamin C, magnesium, and zinc. Most of us, too, aren't able to always eat healthy or even have consistent access to nutrient-rich foods. Finally, for some nutrients like probiotics, no matter how much yogurt, kimchi, or sauerkraut we eat, we may not get enough to do the job, as I explain in a moment.

For these reasons, I believe everyone (with the approval of a practitioner) should consider taking four dietary supplements every day. These four supplements include (1) the marine omega-3 fatty acids EPA and DHA, (2) vitamin D_3, (3) probiotics, and (4) a high-quality multivitamin that includes the B vitamins, selenium, and iodine. These four supplements are what I call "human fertilizer"; we need the nutrients they contain to sustain and optimize our health. In this sense, my human-fertilizer formula is like a good plant fertilizer: while you can grow a plant without one, if you sprinkle on a nutrient-rich fertilizer, your plant will be more likely to thrive, even if it's potted in poor soil or doesn't receive all the light or water it needs.

For supplements to work, they need to be of high quality, which means they follow good manufacturing practices (GMPs) and have been third-party-tested for purity and efficacy. Otherwise, because dietary supplements aren't regulated by the FDA, it's hard to really know what's inside; some supplements may not even contain the nutrients listed on the label, while others may contain too much of them. Many products also have unnecessary additives, including fillers, artificial colors, and even known toxins like lead, mercury, PCBs, talc, and titanium dioxide.[49]

For these reasons, I advise patients to buy only medical- or pharmaceutical-grade supplements, which are held to the same purity standards as prescription drugs. Medical-grade supplements must adhere to GMPs and be third-party-tested for purity and efficacy; contain less than 1 percent binders, fillers, and other inactive ingredients; and offer the most bioavailable form of a nutrient, meaning the one best absorbed by the body. To find medical-grade supplements, though, you need to do some research (see appendix 5 for online supplement resources). Find the websites for manufacturers that claim to be pharmaceutical or medical grade, then look at their third-party test results, and make sure their products contain a USP-Verified Mark, meaning the nonprofit US Pharmacopeia (USP), which is an independent, scientific nonprofit organization, has verified that the product contains the ingredients listed on the label. You can also call a brand for verification and visit any links to third-party test sites on its website for proof of quality.

While medical-grade supplements tend to cost more than regular supplements, I'd rather spend $60 for something that works than $20 on a bottle that may not even have the active nutrient, has a diluted amount, or worse, contains toxins. Talk to your provider about medical-grade supplements: Many healthcare offices sell them or can refer you to a mail-order source, where you may receive discount pricing. I don't recommend buying medical-grade supplements from Amazon, whose suppliers sometimes offer fake versions of real brands (knockoffs) made by overseas manufacturers; they just copy and use the popular brand labeling sold in the United States. Remember that supplements bought online may also be exposed to high heat in storage or transport that can degrade their nutrient quality. Some companies test supplements and share their findings, like Consumer Lab, which can help you find safe, high-quality supplements, although many require a paid annual subscription.

Finally, you need to take supplements regularly and consistently for at least three months to reap their benefits. Like most lifestyle changes, supplementation is not an overnight fix; it's a sustainable habit that can gradually and effectively transform your health.

As always, speak with a healthcare provider before taking any supplements: Some may interact with prescription drugs or may not be advisable for those with existing medical conditions.

THE FOUR HUMAN FERTILIZER SUPPLEMENTS

Omega-3 fatty acids (EPA and DHA). The omega-3 fatty acids EPA and DHA, found primarily in cold-water seafood like salmon, mackerel, tuna, herring, and sardines, are essential for human health, helping control inflammation in the body and brain, improve sleep, aid in weight management, and even prevent chronic disease like cancer, diabetes, heart disease, and Alzheimer's. In fact, a recent study found that people with the highest levels of DHA in the blood had a 17 percent lower risk of all-cause mortality from serious illnesses like cancer and cardiovascular disease.[50] In addition to being anti-inflammatory, these marine fats have detoxifying properties, with studies showing they may help offset the effects of air pollution,[51] bisphenol A (BPA),[52] and a handful of other environmental toxins.

Why not just get your marine omega-3s from cold-water seafood? You certainly can, but up to 95 percent of Americans don't—and our body can't produce EPA and DHA on its own.[53] That's why I recommend taking a high-quality supplement that contains at least 1,000 milligrams combined of EPA and DHA per day; people with inflammatory conditions like arthritis, cancer, or heart disease may want to take up to a total of 3,000 milligrams of EPA plus DHA daily.

Quality matters significantly with omega-3 supplements, since many can contain ocean contaminants and/or toxic metals and/or are rancid, with a recent study finding that most EPA/DHA supplements sold on store shelves had gone bad.[54] For these reasons, choose only brands with third-party test results or medical-grade omega-3 products, and keep the bottle tightly closed to reduce the likelihood of oxidation.

If you're vegan and are avoiding fish-based products altogether, consider taking a high-quality plant-based EPA/DHA supplement made from algae, which contains plant-based EPA and DHA, or flax seeds, which contain the plant-based omega-3 fat alpha-linolenic acid (ALA). While your body can convert a small percentage of ALA to EPA and DHA, know that it's only a modest amount and may not be enough to provide optimal benefits.[55]

Vitamin D. Vitamin D is a hormone, not a vitamin, that helps control how cells and organs function. Among its many benefits, vitamin D has been shown to reduce oxidative stress, protect the brain, regulate immune system function, reduce cancer risk, improve cardiovascular function, lower inflammation, promote autophagy (the removal of unnecessary or dysfunctional cellular parts), slow cellular aging, and remove toxins from the body.[56] To get these advantages, look for vitamin D_3, the most bioavailable form of the nutrient. While some foods like fatty fish and eggs contain vitamin D, most people don't consume these foods in great enough quantities often enough to achieve optimal levels. The body can also manufacture vitamin D from sunlight, but for those of us who don't live near the Equator, which includes much of the contiguous United States, we can't get enough sunlight year-round to make enough vitamin D. Our absorption of vitamin D is also blocked by sunscreen, which is critical to reduce the risk of skin cancer.[57]

If you choose to supplement, consider taking 1,000 to 2,000 IU of vitamin D_3 daily. For best results, have your vitamin D levels checked before you begin to supplement and again every six to twelve months afterward (the blood test for vitamin D, known as 25-hydroxy vitamin D, is covered by most health insurance policies). Liquid vitamin D_3, which is best taken under the tongue, or sublingually, may be better absorbed than capsules—just be sure to check the dropper size and dosing to avoid taking too much.

Pro tip: Vitamin D_3 is one of four fat-soluble vitamins that are stored in the body's fat cells, as opposed to vitamin C and the B vitamins, which are water soluble and not stored in the cells, meaning you pee them out eventually. Because D_3 is fat soluble and stored by the body, if you forget to take the supplement one day, you can double up on the dose the following day, which will prevent any drop in D_3 blood levels.[58]

By comparison, you should aim to take water-soluble vitamins daily, since your body can't store them and doubling the dose the following day won't make up for a missed vitamin the day before.

Multivitamins. In my opinion, taking a high-quality multivitamin is one of the best ways to ensure you have the proper foundation for your health. To achieve this effect, any multivitamin you take should: (1) not contain any added preservatives, coloring, artificial flavoring, or fillers; (2) be third-party-tested for purity and efficacy (visit a company's website and call for verification if you're unsure); and (3) contain all the B vitamins, magnesium, selenium, and 150 mcg of iodine (as sodium iodide), in addition to other nutrients.

Why single out iodine? Many of us don't get enough of this essential mineral ever since American manufacturers in the 1920s stopped fortifying bread and most forms of table salt with iodine.[59] Many of us now use sea salt or Himalayan pink salt for cooking, both of which rarely contain iodine. What's more, many chemicals in our food, water, and personal-care products interfere with iodine absorption. That's a problem, since the mineral is critical to thyroid function. Too much iodine can be harmful, though, so if you have or suspect you have a thyroid issue, speak with a healthcare provider before supplementing. And ignore anyone who tells you there is no research that multivitamins do anything in the body: One recent study of more than twenty thousand older Americans, for example, found that supplementing with a daily multivitamin for at least two years significantly improved memory.[60]

Probiotics. Probiotic supplements are like multivitamins for the gut, helping to replace the healthy microbes we lose every day owing to environmental exposure, emotional stress, nutrient-poor foods, contaminated drinking water, and other factors of daily life. Supplementing with certain probiotic strains may also help the body eliminate

BPA[61] and phthalates, per the research,[62] because good bacteria have a negative charge, allowing them to attract and neutralize metals like lead, cadmium, and mercury, which carry a positive charge (positive and negative charges attract). Probiotics work in the body similar to how microbes work in bioremediation, a technique that uses bacteria and other microorganisms to clean up Superfund sites and toxic waste dumps. I recommend taking at least 20 billion colony-forming units (CFU) daily of a high-quality probiotic supplement that contains several different healthful strains, such as *Lactobacillus* and *Bifidobacterium*. Both refrigerated and shelf-stable probiotics can be effective; what matters more is finding a high-quality, third-party-tested brand. The only hiccup is that shelf-stable brands sold by some online retailers, big-box stores, and vitamin shops may have been exposed to high heat during transport, killing vulnerable microbes, so research the products carefully.

TWO BONUS SUPPLEMENTS I TAKE EVERY DAY

Curcumin. Unless you like turmeric and cook with the spice often, it can be challenging to consume an advantageous amount of curcumin, the active compound in turmeric that is extremely beneficial to both overall health and detoxification pathways. That's why I recommend taking a high-quality curcumin supplement with piperine, the active compound in black pepper that increases absorption of the nutrient by up to 2,000 percent. (If you have any history of liver disease or gastrointestinal troubles, speak with your healthcare provider before taking this supplement.) Start by taking 500 milligrams of curcumin once daily, then increase gradually to 500 milligrams up to four times a day (2,000 mg total).

For some people, taking turmeric at higher doses can increase abdominal discomfort, so if you experience any stomach troubles, titrate down to one or two doses per day. Just be sure to purchase a supplement that's third-party-tested for purity, as curcumin is often harvested from plants grown overseas, where soil pollutants and improper manufacturing practices may lead to contamination with heavy metals like chromium, lead, and mercury.

NAC. As you now know, glutathione is one of the most powerful antioxidants for liver detoxification and overall health. While glutathione supplements exist, they are often pricey and inconvenient, as high-quality forms of the antioxidant usually need to be sold as gels or pastes to increase their absorption by the body. If you want to support and increase the body's levels of glutathione, I recommend supplementing instead with n-acetyl-cysteine (NAC), which contains the amino acid cysteine, one of the three building blocks that make up glutathione. For optimal results, take 500 milligrams of NAC one to two times daily.

In short, eating clean doesn't only mean avoiding foods with toxins; you are also adding in specific healthy foods that can help your body better detoxify, while increasing your nutritional sufficiency. I also believe that taking certain supplements can help improve your body's ability to eliminate environmental toxins.

Chapter 8 Takeaways

- Aim to eat two to five cups (raw or cooked) of cruciferous vegetables daily, such as broccoli, arugula, cauliflower, and kale, as well as alliums (onions, garlic, leeks, chives) daily or as often as possible, all which help activate the liver's most effective phase of detoxification.
- Prioritize consuming good sources of glutathione, such as avocado, asparagus, green beans, cucumber, papaya, and spinach. Additionally, look to consume foods high in cysteine—one of three amino acids found in glutathione—such as cow's dairy, chicken and pork, wheat germ, lentils, oatmeal, eggs, and sunflower seeds.
- As often as possible, eat foods that contain the antioxidant quercetin, the trace mineral selenium, and the spice turmeric to better eliminate toxins, improve nutritional sufficiency, and lower physical stress on a cellular level.
- Look online and in appendix 4 for recipes using artichokes and dandelions (the latter which is an edible herb!) to actively help support your liver and speed detoxification.
- Identify which two days per week are best for you to practice intermittent fasting (if approved by your healthcare provider) to help slow cellular aging, activate cellular cleaning, and speed up the detoxifying enzymes and processes.
- Shop today for my four "human fertilizer" supplements and take them daily: omega-3 fatty acids, vitamin D_3, probiotics, and a multivitamin. I believe everyone needs

outside help to gain nutritional sufficiency, despite how healthy they may eat (check with your healthcare provider before starting any new supplement routine). Just be sure that when you shop, you look for high-quality brands and use the tips and information outlined in this chapter and in the online supplement resources in appendix 5.

CHAPTER 9

The Three Ss to Detoxify

MASSIMO WAS TIRED. Really tired. And he didn't understand why. Sure, owning a pizza parlor on the Jersey Shore wasn't an easy gig, but his father, grandfather, and great-great-grandfather had all done it before him, serving up the family's famous pie without ever complaining. So, why was the fifty-five-year-old having so much trouble keeping his eyes open at work and his body in motion for at least eight hours a day? Was there something seriously wrong with him? Massimo didn't know, which is why and how he ended up in my office.

Massimo wasn't a new patient. I'd seen him in the past for other ailments, which is how he already knew to filter his water, use mostly clean personal-care products, and prioritize eating organic whenever he could. But while Massimo was ahead of the game with these measures, what he didn't know was that his environmental exposure was still high because of a surprising source: pizza boxes. As you might remember from chapter 5, pizza boxes and other forms of greaseproof packaging can contain PFAS, and while pizza boxes aren't necessarily a problem for people who infrequently eat pizza, Massimo was handling these boxes all day long, nearly every day.

What's more, Massimo had another significant source of environmental exposure. Ever since he'd kicked his diet soda habit, he'd started drinking a ton of calorie-free seltzer, which usually contains bisphenol A (BPA) when sold in an aluminum can.

When Massimo came to see me, I didn't immediately assume environmental toxins were to blame for his fatigue. As an integrative doctor, I look carefully and comprehensively at all aspects of a patient's health, including what I can assess during a medical exam and what I can measure with blood work. Additionally, I consider other facets of their life and lifestyle, like any family history of illness, prescription drug use, daily diet, relaxation habits, exercise routine, and so on. At the same time, I always consider environmental exposure because it can play a big role in causing or exacerbating some symptoms and conditions. It's an area that most doctors overlook, which can leave patients struggling for years before they eventually discover what's causing them to feel poorly.

For Massimo, I first took a comprehensive traditional and environmental history of his health while also giving him a full physical exam. That's when I discovered his blood pressure was higher than it had been at his last office visit. I ran basic blood work to test his levels of cholesterol, glucose, white blood cells, and other markers that could indicate an infection or other problem if elevated. I also asked that we do a full thyroid panel and check for antinuclear antibodies (ANA), which if elevated can suggest an autoimmune condition. And while I wouldn't immediately do this for all patients, I recommended we test Massimo's blood for PFAS and his urine for BPA, given his chronic exposure to both toxins.

Thankfully, most of Massimo's blood work that would have suggested other causes of his fatigue, including nutritional, rheumatologic, hormonal, and infectious factors, came back normal. But his PFAS levels were high—above the ninety-fifth percentile of all participants measured nationally. His BPA urinary levels were also elevated; and similar to his blood pressure, his cholesterol was higher than the last time I had seen him, which made sense. High levels of PFAS, BPA, and a handful of other synthetic chemicals can raise both blood pressure and cholesterol. Either way, what Massimo's blood work told me was that environmental toxins were likely playing a role in his fatigue.

To treat the symptom of fatigue, I told Massimo that he first needed to reduce his points of exposure. While PFAS and BPA are pervasive in food, water, furniture, clothing, home goods, and other everyday items, I suggested Massimo focus on his top two sources of exposure that were likely contributing the most and that he could also control: pizza boxes and canned seltzer. I recommended he start wearing latex or nitrile gloves whenever handling the pizza boxes, and instead of spending money on canned seltzer, that he consider switching to filtered water or filtered water mixed with a small amount of his favorite juice—and even a pinch of sea salt or Himalayan pink salt to add electrolytes, as carbonated drinks can increase dehydration. (For an easy-to-make, high-electrolyte beverage, see my recipe for a nontoxic sports drink on page 326.) If he craved seltzer, I suggested he invest in a soda machine that would carbonate the filtered water, which he could drink and store in glass or stainless steel bottles.

In lieu of selling his pizza parlor, however, Massimo would have to do more than reduce his points of exposure. He would also have to work to increase his body's ability to detoxify. That is something nearly all of us, no matter who we are or what we do for work, need to do to reduce our toxic load and improve how we feel. That's because nearly all of us can't avoid exposure to PFAS, BPA, and other environmental toxins. These chemicals are ubiquitous in the air we breathe, the water we drink, the food we consume, and many other items we encounter every day. Chapter 8 discussed how the right foods can improve your body's ability to detoxify and provide the nutritional sufficiency you need to counteract environmental chemicals. In this chapter, we look at the three other most effective ways to strengthen the body's detoxification pathways: (1) by sweating through exercise; (2) sleeping the right way (more quality *and* quantity sleep); and (3) stressing less by actively practicing a technique to reduce anxiety. These three detoxifying powerhouses are what I call the Three Ss.

In Massimo's case, he wasn't exercising regularly because he assumed that being on his feet all day was enough physical activity. But no matter how much we may be on our feet for work or family time, we need sustained, targeted aerobic exercise. Studies recommend a total of at least 150 minutes of *moderate* aerobic activity, like brisk walking, biking, or swimming, per week; or a total of at least 75 minutes of *vigorous* aerobic activity, like running, heavy yard work, or aerobic dancing per week. This movement helps adequately increase the body's immune function, lower inflammation, reduce stress, and maximize the detoxification pathways. While any activity you get will boost your overall health, start-and-stop physical activity undertaken for work, or when you're doing burdensome chores or watching rowdy children, can trigger more stress than it reduces, sparking inflammation and lowering immune function.

As for sleep, while Massimo was spending at least seven hours in bed per night, he had trouble waking up nearly every morning—an indicator that his sleep quality was poor. One of the many problems associated with poor sleep quality is that it will impair the brain's detoxification process. As for stress? Massimo's best way to beat anxiety was with a nightly glass of whisky, which while not entirely unhealthy for most people, wasn't doing his body's detoxification processes any favors.

For busy people like Massimo, finding the time to work out, get better sleep, *and* do something to manage stress isn't always possible. And that's okay. You don't need to work on improving all Three Ss at the same time to improve your body's ability to detoxify. As I told Massimo, identifying the S that's easiest for you to improve or for which you may be the most deficient (if you're averaging only six hours of sleep per night, for example, or you're entirely sedentary) can go a long way toward optimizing your body's detoxification pathways. That's because improving any one S has an additive effect: starting to exercise, for example, or exercising more regularly will boost your sleep quality and help lower your stress levels.[1] Similarly, actively taking steps to manage your stress can also help you sleep better, while giving you the energy or motivation to work out. Think about that for a moment. When you work to improve just one of the Three Ss, you can help boost one, if not both, of the other two.

With Massimo, the easiest S for him to improve upon was exercise. The only reason he hadn't exercised in years was that he believed he didn't have the time to go to the gym. He had joined in the past, only to quit a few weeks later—which was a big waste of money, in his opinion. But as I told him, you don't have to join a gym to exercise. What's more, physical activity has to be enjoyable and easily assimilated into your everyday schedule in order to be sustainable.

With these criteria in mind, Massimo and I brainstormed ways he could exercise that would be both enjoyable and readily sustainable in his daily routine. One easy way was for him to bike to and from work, which wouldn't add a ton of time to his commute. For variety's sake, or when it was too cold to bike, he could walk briskly to work while listening to his favorite podcast; walking would take more time, but because exercise has been shown to increase focus while slashing fatigue, he could make up for any "lost" time by realizing the productivity gains from improved energy and concentration during the day. On weekends, he could play basketball or tennis with his sons, which would be a double win: he'd be able to exercise while also spending quality time with his family.

Three months later, when I saw Massimo again, he told me his fatigue had subsided considerably. He had more energy during the day and was also sleeping better at night. This happened even though he hadn't made any changes other than starting to exercise, avoiding canned seltzer, and wearing gloves at work when possible. During our visit, we also tested his PFAS and BPA levels again, and both were lower—not normal yet, but significantly better than they had been earlier.

Encouraged by his progress and motivated to get his lab results back into a healthy range, Massimo kept up with the exercise, seltzer making, and glove wearing. When I saw him again for a six-month follow-up, his PFAS, BPA, blood pressure, and cholesterol were all normal. More notably, the chronic fatigue he had suffered from for years had vanished. Moreover, he accomplished all this without prescription drugs or sweeping lifestyle changes. Instead, he decreased two sources of exposure while boosting his body's ability to detoxify.

IF YOU PICKED up this book, I'm guessing you have some idea how important regular exercise, high-quality sleep, and stress management are to your overall health. But what most people don't realize is that these actions also strengthen and speed the body's built-in detoxifying processes. In other words, they help reduce the body's burden—the concentration of chemicals currently in the body—and prevent, ease, or treat a range of symptoms, whether toxin-related or due to a specific condition.

In this chapter, we look at the surprising ways in which exercise, sleep, and stress management help optimize the body's detoxification pathways. Knowledge here is key. When I explain to my patients exactly how and why the Three Ss can help them feel better, while preventing or undoing the damage of environmental exposure, they're suddenly more able to make exercise, sleep, and stress management top priorities. In the following pages, you'll learn why and how optimizing your physiology can help maximize how well your body can detoxify, giving you more agency over your health and the chemicals you encounter every day.

How Sweat Helps the Body Detoxify

Exercising regularly is the "single most important thing you can do for your health," according to a report in *Harvard Health*.[2] Being physically active on a regular basis over time has been shown to help prevent and treat disease; spur weight loss; improve critical markers like blood sugar levels, blood pressure, and blood cholesterol; increase lean muscle mass; and prevent and treat mental health issues. In a nutshell, regular exercise improves the function of every system in the body, which in turn improves its ability to detoxify waste, including synthetic toxins. Humans have relied on movement for survival for millions of years, so it makes sense that physical activity is one of the most effective ways to help us detoxify from the effects of our daily living.

At the same time, there are specific ways physical activity helps the body better detoxify. If you're concerned about your environmental exposure, adopting a consistent exercise routine that you enjoy and can sustain is one of the best steps you can take. Not only will you counteract damage, you can also feel more empowered knowing that you're being proactive, which can then reduce any feelings of fear or being overwhelmed that many of us have concerning environmental chemicals. Here are some of the specific ways physical activity helps improve detoxification.

Exercise boosts blood flow. Physical activity increases blood flow in the body, helping to improve its detoxification pathways. Because toxins and other waste products collect in the blood, increased circulation helps the body better filter and eliminate waste by delivering that waste to the top detoxifying organs: the liver, kidneys, gut, lungs, colon, and skin. In particular, improving circulation to the liver—the body's primary filtration system—helps it better clean the blood, convert any toxins into eliminable waste, and speed the metabolism of the nutrients we need to combat the effects of environmental chemicals.[3] (See chapter 7 for more on detoxification.)

Improved blood flow to the liver can also aid in the production of an antioxidant enzyme called *glutathione*, which, as you may remember from chapter 8, plays a critical role in detoxification by helping our cells excrete toxins and even neutralize certain environmental chemicals, like persistent organic pollutants such as PCBs and DDT, turning them into less toxic components.[4] With more blood flow, your body also increases an active group of enzymes in the liver known as *cytochrome P450*, which are able to metabolize environmental chemicals into less toxic compounds that can then be metabolized.[5] Similarly, pumping more blood to the kidneys, lungs, gastrointestinal tract, colon, and skin helps them remove contaminants in the blood more rapidly. Almost any type of physical activity can increase blood flow, including strength training and more restorative types like yoga and tai chi, but aerobic exercise, like walking, running, swimming, biking, and dancing, typically increase blood flow the most.

Exercise improves lymphatic flow. Exercise is one of the most effective ways to increase the function of the lymphatic system, an essential circuit of organs, vessels, and nodes that collect and drain impurities from the cells and tissues. Because the lymphatic system doesn't have a pump like the circulatory system does (that is, the heart), the lymphatic system relies on muscle movement and contraction to move lymph fluid through the body. That fluid then collects toxins and filters them in the lymph nodes before returning them to the bloodstream to be eliminated. Massage, deep breathing, and other therapies have been shown to increase lymphatic drainage, but traditional full-body exercise like walking, running, biking, swimming, yoga, strength training, and Pilates may be more effective, boosting lymphatic flow up to three times higher than when the body is at rest, according to the studies.[6] Physical activity performed in water, like swimming and water aerobics, may boost lymphatic flow, thanks to the pressure from the water.

HOW A TRAMPOLINE CAN HELP YOU DETOX

Trampolines have become a hot health trend in recent years, with more research showing that jumping on a mini-trampoline, also known as *rebounding*, can provide a number of benefits. One of those benefits is increased lymphatic flow, with some scientists estimating that rebounding may boost lymph flow by up to thirty times the normal rate.[7] If you are among those who struggle to find the time or motivation to exercise, or simply don't think traditional forms of physical activity are fun, you may want to consider investing in a mini-trampoline. Prices vary, but you can find one online for as little as $60.

According to the research, rebounding doesn't feel like exercise to many people, but at the same time, a nineteen-minute workout on a mini-trampoline can burn as many calories as running six miles an hour on flat ground for the same amount of time, per one study. Using a mini-trampoline may also improve balance and pelvic-floor function, which can increase pleasure during sex, help treat urinary incontinence and constipation, and prevent pelvic-floor prolapse.[8] Given the newfound popularity of rebounding, there are now lots of online videos that can help you learn to use a mini-trampoline safely and effectively to get a good workout.

Exercise boosts immune system function. The stronger your immune system, the better able your body is to fight off environmental toxins. Exercise strengthens the immune system in a number of ways, in part by stimulating the flow of lymph, which is part of the immune system. At the same time, exercise increases the production of both immune cells and cytokines,[9] the latter being signaling proteins that help direct the immune system to fight infection, cancerous cells, and foreign substances in the body, like synthetic chemicals. Regular exercise also reduces chronic inflammation,[10] helping to ease or treat symptoms associated with the condition like fatigue, joint pain, insomnia, depression, anxiety, GI issues, and weight gain. Just twenty minutes of moderate exercise performed consistently over time may be all you need to reduce the blood markers of inflammation, according to the research.[11]

Exercise improves the variety and quantity of healthy gut bacteria. The healthier your gut microbiome, the better able your body is to detoxify and neutralize or minimize harmful environmental toxins. Today, mounting research shows that exercise helps increase the quantity of healthy bacteria and by-products in the gut, while decreasing the amounts of unhealthy, pro-inflammatory bacteria. This is one reason why athletes have greater gut diversity than do sedentary people.[12]

Exercise burns fat and lowers insulin resistance. Certain environmental toxins, like PCBs, pesticides, dioxins, and flame retardants, are stored in fat cells, which means the more fat you have, the more chemicals your body can accumulate.[13] (The same is true of the fish and animals we eat, which is why removing fat from seafood and meat before cooking or consuming it can help reduce chemical intake.) Adopting a consistent exercise routine over time decreases adipose tissue, thereby lowering the body's ability to stockpile environmental toxins. Physical activity, especially strength training, also increases lean muscle mass and improves insulin resistance. Insulin resistance occurs when the body can't properly process insulin, a fat-storing hormone that, in excess, can lead to the development of diabetes. Improving insulin resistance has a multitude of benefits, including the ability to boost gut, brain, liver, and cardiovascular health, all of which bolster the body's detoxification pathways.

Because exposure to environmental chemicals may cause insulin resistance, according to the research,[14] exercising to improve the body's ability to process the hormone can mitigate the effect. One study, in fact, showed that people with diabetes who exercise regularly increased the type of gut bacteria shown to improve insulin resistance.[15]

Exercise improves sleep quality and quantity. Regular physical activity improves not only how much sleep we get (sleep quantity) but also the quality of that sleep, which is critical.[16] While some of us like Massimo may spend seven hours or more in bed every night, the sleep we get may not be restorative, for various reasons. Chronic health conditions, caffeine and alcohol use, and too much stress or anxiety, among other factors, can sabotage sleep quality, impairing how well your brain can clear toxins during the night. But regular exercise can boost both sleep quality and quantity, according to numerous studies, with some research showing that aerobic activity improves sleep as effectively as sleeping pills, without the side effects.[17]

Physically active jobs like Massimo's, on the other hand, don't always promote sleep because the job can add stress and anxiety (exercise reduces both) without necessarily offering the physical benefits that exercise provides. People who work on their feet can even experience joint or muscle aches and pains that can prevent them from falling asleep or staying asleep.[18]

Exercise reduces stress. If you've ever felt elated or as though your problems dissipated after a sweat session, you've experienced the stress-busting effects of exercise. This is one of the best ways to ease anxiety and lower physical, mental, and emotional tensions. Finding a means to manage stress will strengthen the body's detoxification pathways, while counteracting stress itself, which acts like a toxin in the body.

Exercise makes you sweat. Physical activity makes you sweat, which is beneficial for a number of reasons, including that we may be able to sweat out trace amounts of environmental toxins. Researchers have found that human sweat can contain phthalates,[19] PCBs, perfluorinated compounds,[20] certain heavy metals such as arsenic and lead,[21] and BPA.[22] While the jury is still out on whether eliminating trace amounts of toxins through sweat can improve health, I'll take every advantage I can get. For this reason, I actively try to sweat more during exercise, piling on extra layers before I go running, even if it's warm out. I encourage my patients to engage in some sort of sweat-generating activity, whether that's exercising, using a sauna, or walking with extra layers, for at least thirty minutes, five days per week.

What's the absolute best way to exercise to optimize detoxification? There is no one activity in particular that's been proven definitively to increase detoxification. What matters more is sustaining any kind of activity over time, so choose the exercise you like doing the best. Otherwise, if you exercise only sporadically, or for a few weeks or months, you won't reap the benefits. Similarly, if you force yourself to work out in a way you don't enjoy or you must make grave sacrifices to fit the exercise into your schedule, you'll be less likely to reduce stress through exercise, as your workout may cause you more anxiety.

If you haven't found a type of exercise you enjoy, consider alternative forms of activity, like dancing, gardening, or doing a home strengthening routine with push-ups, squats, and/or other bodyweight exercises. As long as the activity raises your heart rate and/or strengthens your muscles, you'll see benefits. If you're dealing with a medical condition, lower-body injury, or mobility issue that prevents you from traditional exercise, talk with your provider to see if chair aerobics may be an option for you; the seated activity can give you a surprisingly good workout, depending on the intensity you choose. To learn more about chair aerobics or for workout ideas, go online to find free video classes.

THE NO-EFFORT WAY TO SWEAT MORE AND STRESS LESS

For centuries, people in Finland, Japan, Iceland, Turkey, and other countries around the world have used saunas to detoxify and boost their overall health. Today, research confirms what many cultures have known all along: that regularly immersing the body in intense dry heat can improve detoxification pathways by increasing blood flow and reducing blood pressure.[23] Studies also show that sauna bathing (as it's sometimes called) can reduce levels of C-reactive protein, the leading marker of systemic (body-wide) inflammation.[24] A systemic review of more than forty clinical studies found that sauna bathing for anywhere from five to twenty minutes in a single session, or multiple sessions totaling thirty minutes or more cumulative time daily, may also be beneficial to immunity-related conditions like rheumatoid arthritis, fibromyalgia, chronic fatigue, and allergic rhinitis. In addition, it may potentially improve the skin's moisture barrier.[25] And you don't need a study to tell you that saunas are relaxing, which helps reduce stress. If you sit in a sauna, you'll also sweat a lot, which can help your body eliminate toxins in trace amounts. I'm such a fan of sauna bathing that I saved money for years to install a tiny one in my home, which I try to use at least once a week.

I want to be clear, though: Saunas don't impart the same degree of detoxifying benefits and overall health impacts that exercise does. You'll also need to make sure you hydrate well with electrolytes before, during, and after a sauna to avoid dehydration, which can undo a sauna's potential health benefits. Finally, if you're pregnant or have a medical condition, speak with your doctor before using a sauna.

How Sleep Helps the Body Detoxify

Walk into any bookstore or browse retailers online, and you'll find hundreds of books extolling the benefits of sleep. But what many authors don't know is just how vital sleep is to our body's ability to detoxify—more specifically, to our brain's ability to detoxify. Sleep is the brain's best time to remove toxins and other waste that build up during the day. When we're asleep, the brain's glymphatic system, similar to the body's lymphatic system, mixes cerebrospinal fluid with interstitial fluid (the fluid that surrounds cells and blood vessels) to wash toxins from the brain. Nearly all this activity occurs while we're asleep, as glymphatic activity drops by a whopping 90 percent when we're awake.[26]

The reason sleep quality is so important to the brain's detoxifying process is that most of its washing and cleaning takes place during deep sleep, or slow-wave sleep, the most restorative stage of the body's four-stage sleep cycle.[27] If you're not getting enough quality sleep, you're also not getting enough deep sleep, which means your brain's glymphatic system has less time to remove toxins.

How to tell if your sleep quality is less than ideal? If you regularly have problems waking up, suffer from daytime drowsiness, feel moody or irritable during the day, and/or are unable to focus despite spending at least seven hours per night in bed, you likely have poor sleep quality.

Working to improve your sleep quality with exercise and stress management—the two additive Ss—can also improve the function of your liver, which is governed by the body's circadian rhythms (its twenty-four-hour sleep-wake cycle).[28] This is one reason why people with poor sleep quality or quantity are more likely to develop liver conditions, including nonalcohol fatty liver disease, the most common chronic liver disease worldwide.[29]

Because I'm a rheumatologist and environmental-health expert, not a sleep scientist, I'm not going to expand on all the ways to get more quality sleep; as I mentioned earlier, there are a ton of books, articles, and blogs on the subject. But I do want to make one point, because amid all the sleep tips and tricks I've heard, not a lot of experts are espousing this one: *good sleep takes work.*

You'll likely need to do some trial and error as you experiment with which habits and circumstances best support your unique body's best sleep outcomes. You will have to make compromises or sacrifices to get ahead. What this means is that you may have to give up going out with friends on some nights, or stream fewer shows, or find a way to put away work for the night to improve your sleep. Additionally, keeping your phone in another room or having that uncomfortable conversation with a partner who snores may be necessary to boost your quality sleep (and theirs). You also might need to invest in blackout shades or pay to run an air conditioner at night, since light pollution and bedroom temperatures above 67 degrees can interfere with optimal sleep.

For those who suffer from frequent sleeplessness or insomnia, review your bedtime habits and reduce your technology use before bed. Avoid any work too close to bedtime, which can create "monkey mind," or a restless, unsettled state. You can also consider a magnesium supplement in glycinate, citrate, and/or L-threonate form in a dose of 200 to 400 milligrams taken before bed. Other types of magnesium, like citrate and oxide, are less effective for sleep and can result in loose stools. Just be sure to consult with your healthcare provider before adding any supplement, especially if you have any type of kidney impairment that might inhibit your body's ability to remove magnesium.

I constantly and consciously make small sacrifices to get more quality sleep. For example, I usually don't attend late-night events or make social plans with other couples past 9 p.m., so as to prioritize my sleep. (I've often found many couples are like-minded and are more than happy to meet my husband and me for dinner at 5:30 p.m.!) I'm willing to do this because I know that when I get enough sleep, my focus, energy, mood, and immunity all improve considerably. Whenever I'm tempted to stay up late watching something on TV or scrolling through social media, I remind myself that my brain will work better and be healthier if I turn off the TV or put my phone away so that I have more time to rest, restore, and detoxify.

How Stress Management Helps the Body Detoxify

Most of us know that stress is unhealthy. But in an age when so many things are identified as being possibly harmful, it can be easy to overlook just how toxic stress is on the body and brain. The truth is, psychological forms of stress like anxiety or depression can be as detrimental to our health as smoking cigarettes or being obese. That's because they increase the risk of heart disease, stroke, arthritis, back pain, and stomach issues as much as cigarettes and obesity can, according to University of California, San Francisco, researchers.[30]

As a doctor, I see stress as another toxic environmental chemical exposure, capable of inflicting the same degree of harm on a body as synthetic toxins can. Too much stress can alter the body's microbiome and increase gut permeability, triggering leaky gut syndrome and boosting the number and speed at which toxins enter the bloodstream.[31] Long-lasting stress can also cause chronic, systemic inflammation and reduce immunity—to the point that stress is believed to cause some autoimmune conditions.[32]

When it comes to environmental exposure, your body will have a difficult time combating chemicals if you're always stressed and not taking active steps to manage it. Stress impairs every physiological system in the body, impacting how well your liver, kidneys, gut, skin, lungs, lymphatic system, glymphatic system, colon, and other organs, tissues, and structures can do their job.

What does it mean to "actively" manage stress? For most of us, telling ourselves that we're simply going to stress less isn't enough. We need to commit time every day, even if it's just five minutes, to do a targeted activity that will help reduce stress and anxiety. This can be as easy as practicing yoga in your home or doing deep-breathing exercises in your office, which can reduce stress and inflammation on a cellular level.[33] Or try progressive muscle relaxation, in which you tense or tighten one muscle group at a time before relaxing to release the tension. There are many other types of stress relief, including painting or drawing, practicing positive self-talk, and engaging in traditional talk or cognitive behavioral therapy with a professional. For many people, meditation is a great way to reduce stress, with studies showing that practicing for just five minutes daily can lower stress.[34] If you're new to meditation or have struggled with the practice in the past, download an app to your smartphone to help guide you.

One way I like to counter stress is by taking warm baths with Epsom salts three to four times per week after work or before bed. Not only does the activity help me pause and separate myself from everything else that happened in my day—seeing patients, managing my kids, running errands—but the Epsom salts have been shown to reduce muscle aches, lessen arthritis symptoms, and improve sleep by reducing excitatory chemicals in the brain.

NOISE POLLUTION: A MAJOR SOURCE OF STRESS FEW DOCTORS TALK ABOUT

Honking cars, airplanes roaring overhead, emergency vehicle sirens, loud music in restaurants and retail shops, and people streaming their videos in public places: We're constantly assaulted by noise pollution, which is any unwanted or disturbing sound. While most people don't think twice about noise pollution, research shows that it's a serious problem for our health because it increases our stress hormones and levels of inflammation.[35]

Noise pollution can also spark activity in the amygdala, a structure in the brain associated with fear and pain. Among other concerns, exposure to chronic noise pollution may act as an *obesogen*, a compound that promotes weight gain, by disrupting the body's circadian rhythms and interfering with the metabolism.[36] Chronic noise pollution has also been shown to cause or worsen heart disease, type 2 diabetes, mental health problems, sleep disorders, and cognitive issues like memory impairment and attention deficits.[37] Noise pollution is such a threat to human health that the Environmental Protection Agency (EPA) calls it a "growing danger to the health and welfare of the Nation's people."[38] According to one study that cites the World Health Organization, approximately 1.5 million years of healthy life are lost annually in Western Europe alone because of its traffic noise.[39]

If you're curious how loud your home, office, or other environment is, you can measure the noise levels using an inexpensive handheld sound decibel meter or download a decibel app to your phone. Just know that all devices and apps vary in quality and degree of sensitivity, so be sure to read any reviews of them and contact the manufacturer for additional information.

If you're constantly around noise and want to improve your body's detoxification pathways, consider targeted steps to reduce that noise pollution. Even if you're not consciously bothered by noise pollution, research shows that your body still initiates stress responses whenever you're surrounded by unwanted sound.[40]

The following steps can limit your exposure to noise pollution and help optimize your body's detoxification processes:

- Wear noise-canceling or noise-reducing earplugs or headphones in loud areas.
- Invest in soundproof shades, blinds, curtains, or window treatments, especially in your bedroom if noise pollution is interfering with your sleep.
- Download a white-noise app to your smartphone or purchase a white-noise machine that plays nature sounds or other soft, relaxing noises that can help mask disturbing sounds.
- Plant shrubs and trees around your home, which absorb sound and can cut noise by up to 10 decibels.[41]
- Consider installing special insulation, thicker materials in walls, and hardwood floors if you're remodeling or building a home.
- Use soft wall hangings and area rugs to help absorb sound at home.

Chapter 9 Takeaways

- Start exercising more by making a list of the activities you like and engaging in one, or by trying a new type of physical activity if you're tired of your current routine. Remember that anything that gets you moving, including aerobic exercise, strength training, weight lifting, and restorative activity like yoga and tai chi, can help your body better detoxify in a number of ways. (Be sure to speak with your doctor before adopting a greater degree of physical activity.)

- Aim to get at least 150 minutes of moderate aerobic activity, like brisk walking, biking, or swimming, per week or at least 75 minutes of vigorous aerobic activity, like running, heavy yard work, and aerobic dancing, per week, which will help increase immune function, lower inflammation, reduce stress, and maximize your body's detoxification pathways.

- Take the time now to assess and identify factors that may be interfering with the quality or quantity of your sleep, then strategize some solutions. Are you staying out too late and not getting home in time to get at least seven hours shut-eye per night? If so, you may need to refuse more evening events or meet friends or family at an earlier hour. If your bedroom is too hot, bright, or noisy, consider running the A/C or investing in blackout shades or a white-noise app or machine. Are you waking up frequently in the middle of the night with anxiety or thinking about all the things you have to do? Take time during the day to practice stress management, and limit work and screen time before bed to prevent the racing thoughts that can prevent sleep or wake you up later.

- Look online for an inexpensive mini-trampoline and start rebounding daily to increase lymphatic drainage and overall detox!
- If approved by your healthcare provider, find a local gym or fitness center with a sauna and go as often as possible, for up to twenty minutes per session, being sure to hydrate adequately with filtered water afterward.
- Find just five minutes today to perform any type of active stress management, like meditation, yoga, or deep breathing exercises; this tiny duration of time (shorter than some people stand in line waiting for a morning coffee) can help reduce anxiety and ease psychological tension.

THE *DETOXIFY* PLAN
Twenty-One Days to Restore and Improve Your Health

CONGRATULATIONS! AFTER READING those nine chapters, you're now a de facto expert in how environmental toxins affect the body; where and how they hide in our food, water, home, and personal products; and what you can do to reduce your exposure while increasing your body's ability to detoxify. Because there's so much information in this book, it can be a lot to process and implement, which is why I created this 21-Day Plan. It's designed to help you apply all the tips, tricks, and scientific knowledge you've gleaned to one easy, actionable three-week scheme. At the end of three weeks, you can expect to feel more energetic, optimistic, clear-headed, lighter, and leaner, while experiencing a possible reduction in any troubling symptoms.

Before you start, here are nine key things to know about the next twenty-one days:

1. Always speak with your doctor before starting any plan that includes new dietary supplements and nutritional and exercise habits. Continue to take all medications as prescribed.
2. Take the time to read through the entire plan before you dive in, as it can require time, preparation, and planning.
3. For best results, follow the "four As" (Assess, Avoid, Add, Allow) in that order, *assessing* your exposure so you know which exposure points to *avoid*, then *adding* new elements like detoxifying foods and supplements before *allowing* a new mindset (for a refresher on the "four As," see page ix).
4. Don't dismiss the small stuff. Even seemingly minor changes to your regular habits, especially when you maintain them over time, can bring big results.
5. Know that you may experience temporary symptoms, such as headaches, lightheadedness, diarrhea, cramps, bloating, body aches, fatigue, and mood changes, as your body detoxifies. These are most often due to new dietary or lifestyle changes, reflecting the increased mobilization of toxins out of the body. If the symptoms persist or are severe, speak with a medical practitioner.
6. Drink plenty of filtered water throughout the twenty-one days to help your body better eliminate toxins and stay hydrated. If you struggle to drink plain water or want to increase your hydration by adding electrolytes, consider making my nontoxic electrolyte drink (page 326).
7. Feel empowered to modify the plan to fit your individual needs. Check in with yourself regularly to assess if an aspect, such as intermittent fasting, isn't working for you. Keep in mind, though, that experiencing growing pains is normal whenever you adopt healthier habits. Eating healthier, exercising more frequently, and making small sacrifices to prioritize your quality and quantity of sleep all require efforts that are well worth the rewards.

8. Remember that reducing your exposure to toxins is a journey, not a destination. To this day, I continue to make changes to my habits and surroundings. You will find some strategies listed in the next few pages that will click right away, while others may take you longer to adapt to. What's important, especially if you are feeling overwhelmed, frightened, or furious, is to remember that the *power to change your environment is in your hands.*

9. Curiosity is your greatest weapon, so channel the concern I know you already have for your health into curiosity about your surroundings, your diet and other daily habits, and your indoor and outdoor environments. Ask questions. Don't be afraid to experiment with different strategies. And use trial and error to find the lifestyle changes that work best for you, your family, and your pets.

THE FIRST FEW days of this plan are dedicated to assessing and identifying possible exposure sources of chemicals in your diet, personal-care products, and home and work environment, and any symptoms that may be related to them. Once you know your exposure sources and/or the symptoms you want to treat, you can begin to strategically attack them by avoiding or replacing those items in your water, daily diet, personal-care routine, and home or office that may be increasing your toxin load and/or causing or aggravating symptoms.

After you start reducing your chemical exposure, you can ramp up your body's ability to detoxify by focusing on the Three Ss—Sweat, Sleep, and Stress. (Otherwise, trying to boost your natural detoxification pathways while you're still exposed to an abundance of dietary and environmental toxins can be counterproductive.)

When you finish the 21-Day Plan, allow yourself to begin cultivating a new mindset that will help you make these changes a permanent part of your life.

Week One: Assess

Before you make any changes to your diet, lifestyle habits, and/or home, use the first seven days of the twenty-one-day plan to gather some hard data on your biggest exposure points. That way, you know what to avoid and how to personalize your program to get the most bang for your buck. Once you're able to identify your primary points of exposure, you will be well on your way to keeping them from even entering your body in the first place.

So, for this first week, take the time to sit down and complete the following three surveys: (1) 50-Question Health and Body Survey, (2) Symptom Evaluation Survey, and (3) Home and Workplace Survey.

For scoring:

> <5: You're doing things well but could make a few tweaks to your lifestyle routine.
>
> <15: Good job, but keep working on reducing your chemical exposures.
>
> >30: You likely have a high body burden of toxic chemicals, and there is no better time than now to reduce your exposure.

Note: The Symptom Evaluation Worksheet (beginning on page 267) can help you evaluate whether your symptoms change during and after the 21-Day Plan. To complete the worksheet, rate your symptoms over time on a scale from 1 to 10, with 1 = no symptom and 10 = acute symptom.

Additionally, at the start of the 21-Day Plan, you might want to *consider laboratory testing*. If you're thinking of having any blood or urine analysis done, the best time to do so is during Week One. That way, you can make it part of your assessment work so you have baseline readings for your nutrient and toxin levels (see Appendix 2, Medical and Other

Laboratory Testing). If you have the resources, repeat those tests in three to six months' time, after you're able to implement and maintain the new habits. That will help you determine how your nutrient and toxin levels have changed. Remember that you may have to be your own patient advocate; ask your primary-care doctor to retest at the intervals you want.

50-Question Health and Body Survey can help you determine the degree of chemicals entering your body:

No = 0, Yes = 1 point

Food and Drink

Do you regularly drink water from a well or municipal tap? _____
Do you filter your drinking water? __1__
Do you regularly eat processed foods? _____
Do you regularly eat conventionally grown fruit and vegetables? _____
Do you drink soda (diet or regular)? _____
Do you use Splenda, Equal, or other artificial sweeteners? _____
Do you regularly eat large seafood like tuna, swordfish, or lobster? _____
Do you eat farm-raised salmon? __1__
Are you taking three or more supplements daily? __1__
Do you consume alcohol or caffeine in excess? _____

Personal Care and Cleaning

Do you use scented perfume, musk, or body spray? __1__
Do you wear antiperspirant? _____
Do you use more than ten personal care products daily that contain known toxins? _____
Do you use air fresheners, plug-ins, or scented candles in your home? __1__
Do you use cleaning and/or laundry products with chemical names listed in the ingredients? _____
Do you dust and vacuum your home less than once a week? __1__
Do you *not* read the ingredient list of personal-care products before you buy them? __1__

Home Furnishing, Bedding, and Air Quality

Do you smoke, vape, or live with a smoker? _____
Do you use stain-guard chemicals on your couch? _____
Was your couch manufactured before 2013? _____
Do you use "wrinkle-free" bedding? _____
Do you light candles or incense daily or weekly? _____
Do you have gas appliances such as a stove and/or washer/dryer? __1__
Do you wear dry-cleaned clothes? __1__

Cookware and Food Packaging
Do you use nonstick pans and bakeware?   1
Do you use plastic untensils, cups, and/or plates?   1
Do you use a plastic spatula or strainer?   1
Do you eat food microwaved in plastic "steam-in" bags or other?   1
Do you use plastic containers for food and drink storage?   1
Do you get takeout food daily or weekly?
Do you use canned foods daily or weekly?
Do you get takeout coffee in a paper cup?

WiFi Use and Electric and Magnetic Field (EMF) Exposure
Do you sleep with your cell phone next to your head?   1
Do you hold up your cell phone to your ear for most calls?
Do you carry your cell phone in your front pants pocket or in your bra?
Do you place your computer on your lap to do work?

Home and Work Environment
Do you live in or commute daily or weekly to a congested city?
Do you live in a home that contains lead pipes or copper plumbing?   1
Was your home built before 1978?   1
Do you live in a home that has paint dating from the 1970s?   1
Do you live within 1 mile of conventionally farmed land?
Do you have vinyl floor covering?   √
Are you surrounded by artificial light most hours of the day?   1
Do you feel stressed at work or at home most of the time?

Occupational and Other Exposures
Do you work around and/or handle industrial chemicals daily or weekly (paint, solvents, gasoline, pesticides/herbicides, some art materials)?
Do you work as a cosmetician, manicurist, aesthetician, makeup artist, or masseuse?
Do you use and/or store insecticides in your home?
Do you handle cat litter daily or weekly?   1
Do you use flea and tick collars for your pet?
Do you work in a loud environment?   1

Total   2v

Symptom Evaluation Worksheet can help you evaluate whether your symptoms change during and after the 21-Day Plan. To complete the worksheet, rate your symptoms over time on a scale from 1 to 10, 1 being no symptom, 10 being acute symptom. When filling out the worksheet, keep the following in mind:

- The timing of your symptoms after an exposure occurred
- Intensity of symptoms
- Consistency of symptoms
- Other possible exposures that may contribute to symptoms

Symptom	Day 1	Day 7	Day 14	Day 21	Month 6	Month 9	Month 12	Month 18
Abdominal								
Bloating ✓								
Constipation								
Diarrhea								
Pain ✓								
Abnormal periods								
Frequency								
Heavy flow								
Allergy symptoms ✓								
Itchy eyes ✓								
Runny nose ✓								
Sneezing								
Anxiety ✓								
Blood sugar level (if diabetic)								
Brain fog ✓								
Depression								
Fatigue ✓								
Headache								
Infections								
Respiratory								
Skin/cellulitis								
Urinary tract ✓	✓							

Symptom	Day 1	Day 7	Day 14	Day 21	Month 6	Month 9	Month 12	Month 18
Migraine								
Musculoskeletal symptoms								
Joint pain								
Joint swelling								
Muscle pain								
Muscle weakness								
Shortness of breath								
Skin changes								
Dryness								
Eczema								
Psoriasis								
Rash								
Rosacea								
Tremors								
Weight gain								
Weight loss								

Home and Workplace Worksheet can help you identify the toxic exposures in your home and workplace so that you can work toward removing them. To complete the worksheet, consider each item on the list, putting a check next to those to which you are exposed:

Indoor air quality

- [x] Windows that are most often closed (unless you live in a city or near conventionally farmed land)
- [x] Few to no green plants inside
- [ ] HVAC system without regular or recent filter changes
- [ ] Air filter without regular or recent filter changes
- [ ] Humidifier without regular or recent cleaning
- [x] Gas stove and appliances
- [ ] Synthetic air fresheners
- [ ] Synthetic bug sprays
- [ ] Flea and tick spray for pets
- [x] Synthetic or perfumed litter used for cats or other small animals
- [x] Scented candles
- [x] Incense
- [x] Wood smoke

Conventional cleaning products including:
- [x] Surface cleaner
- [x] Dish soap
- [ ] Dishwasher soap
- [ ] Window cleaner
- [x] Carpet powder
- [x] Laundry detergent
- [ ] Fabric softener
- [x] Floor cleaner (e.g., Swiffer, Mr. Clean)
- [x] Toilet bowl cleaner
- [ ] Shower cleaner
- [ ] Oven cleaner
- [ ] Drain cleaner
- [ ] Scented trash bags

Construction and renovations including:
- [ ] Demolition
- [ ] Cleanup
- [ ] New paint
- [ ] New carpeting or flooring

Furniture

- [ ] Couch manufactured before 2013 (or with flame retardants)
- [ ] Synthetic pillows

Flooring

- [ ] Do you remove your shoes at the door?
- [ ] Carpeting
- [ ] Carpet backing
- [x] Synthetic rugs
- [ ] Synthetic flooring

Paint

- [ ] Outdoor paint (before 1978)
- [ ] Indoor paint (before 1978)
- [ ] Paints for hobbies or art projects

Home water

Unfiltered tap water including from:
- ☐ Refrigerator doors
- ☐ Ice cubes
- ☐ Faucet
- ☐ Countertop
- ☐ Showerheads

Outdoor lawn, gardens, and plants

- ☐ Synthetic weed sprays
- ☐ Synthetic pesticides
- ☐ Synthetic fertilizer
- ☐ Artificial turf
- ☐ Wood playgrounds (can contain preservatives with arsenic)

Week Two: Avoid

It's toxin takedown week! This is when you'll begin to remove the most harmful toxins from your daily routine. Here's what to do each day so that you can focus and maximize your time:

Day 8: Use your 50-Question Health and Body Survey to start removing the toxins you put into, on, and around your body.

- Grab a trash bag or cardboard box and remove all the packaged snacks, bottled drinks (including water), condiments, fresh foods like deli meats and conventionally raised meat and dairy products, and any other items you know contain toxins. Package them up to donate to a local food bank or shelter. (While donating isn't always ideal, since it exposes others to toxins, shelters and food banks often buy these items anyway, and donating them can help those institutions save money that they can then use to purchase cleaner foods in the future.)
- Toss out and start avoiding artificial sweeteners (saccharine, aspartame, sucralose) and "natural" nonnutritive sweeteners like stevia and monk fruit. Natural sweeteners such as real honey, pure maple syrup, and molasses are okay to use in small amounts.
- Toss out or avoid seafood that's highest in toxins, including farmed salmon and tilapia, swordfish, Chilean sea bass, and imported shrimp (except from the Netherlands, where the water quality is considered cleaner). See pages 141–42 on how to identify high-toxin seafood.
- Avoid tobacco (first- and secondhand smoke), excessive use of caffeine and alcohol, and recreational drugs. People can tolerate caffeine at varying levels, but excessive use of caffeine is typically considered more than 200 milligrams per day for an adult, or the equivalent of two strong eight-ounce cups of coffee. Excessive drinking, on the other hand, is

defined as four or more drinks on a single occasion, or more than eight drinks per week for women and five or more drinks on a single occasion or more than fifteen drinks per week for men.

- Because food packaging also plays a role in chemical exposure, toss out or avoid foods that have been cooked, served, or stored in plastic, particularly hot foods and drinks. Toss out or avoid canned foods and drinks whenever possible; and toss out or avoid food wrapped or cooked in plastic wrap.

Day 9: Go room to room in your home and collect all the toxic household cleaners you have. Pack them up to be donated to a local animal shelter or other nonprofit. Here are some tips to help you with the process:

- Look up cleaning products on the EWG website or use its Healthy Living app (see page 185) to determine the toxicity, if you're unsure.
- Toss all air fresheners, plug-ins, incense, and candles that haven't been fully vetted for safe ingredients.
- If using a commercial carpet cleaning service, request they steam-clean only without added chemicals.
- Pet owners should avoid pet foods and treats made with artificial ingredients; avoid using cat litter with a fragrance; avoid flea and tick sprays, collars, and topical ointments, swapping them for essential oils that work just as well to control infestation; and avoid plastic chew toys and unfiltered drinking water.

Day 10: Today's the day to toss out those noxious cosmetics and personal-care products! To help determine their toxicity, look up the personal-care products on EWG's Skin Deep database (see page 58) or similar website or app, and toss out those with poor ratings. (Any item that scores 3 or higher gets tossed in my household, while a rating of 2 or below is ideal.) Products to evaluate include the following:

- Shampoos and conditioners; deodorants, aftershave, and bar and hand soaps; face wash and body wash
- Hair gels, mousse, cream, and all other hair styling products
- Contact solutions
- Makeup—eye shadow, foundation, mascara, eyeliner, lip balm, lipstick, etc.
- Face creams, serums, masks, and body lotions
- Cologne, musk, perfume, and fragrances
- Nail polish, polish remover, and other nail products

Feminine-care products often get overlooked, even though any chemicals they contain can be easily absorbed through the tissue of the vaginal canal, so make sure to check your tampons, pads, feminine sprays, and douches for toxicity. Also, consider using fewer personal-care products overall to reduce your exposure to sneaky chemicals.

Day 11: It's another day in the kitchen, but today, focus on getting rid of any toxic cookware. Box up the following to donate to a local food shelter. (Remember that food shelters often have to buy cookware anyway, and if you help them to save money by donating, they may be able to invest in nontoxic cookware in the future.)

- Toss your plastic spatulas, plastic cups, plates, utensils, reusable plastic water bottles, sports bottles, plastic Tupperware, plastic mixing bowls, nonstick pans, bakeware, and cookie sheets.
- Avoid heating any foods or drinks in plastic packaging, opting for stainless steel, cast iron, or heat-resistant glass instead.
- If you must use plastic, avoid storing food or eating from plastic

containers with recycling codes 3, 6, and 7. (Remember, "5, 4, 1, and 2; all the rest are bad for you!")

Day 12: Avoid or toss out the pesticides and industrial toxins that affect the air you breathe:

- Remove insect sprays and other home and personal insecticides.
- Opt for commercial lawn treatment providers who use nontoxic chemicals such as "bio-herbicide," which rely on natural microbes instead of synthetic pesticides. Use lawn and garden products made with vinegar and 100 percent natural oils like eucalyptus or citronella, without synthetic additives. Avoid indoor insect fumigation services.
- Get rid of any industrial chemicals in your closets and garage, including any old, opened, or unused paints, solvents, wood stains, industrial glues, and floor cleaners. (Studies show that homes with attached garages that contain gas or kerosene, gas-powered equipment, and/or lawn-care products have an increased risk of ALS.[1]) Check your local or township municipality for their household hazardous waste disposal days, when you can bring hazardous products to their facility for safe disposal.
- If you have clothes that must be dry-cleaned, identify a service provider that offers all organic options. Remember to leave time to "off-gas" the cleaned clothing outside before bringing it inside your home.
- If you're planning for renovations to your home or a new purchase, select electric appliances over gas ones.

Day 13: Examine your furniture and home furnishings to consider removing any synthetic foam pillows and changing out any toxic mattresses.

- Look for labels that specify a product is made from organic cotton, organic latex rubber, 100 percent cotton, or is GOTS-certified, which means it's been tested for organic fibers.
- Check your couch label to see if it lists toxic flame-retardant chemicals (see page 193) and consider swapping out for a new couch.
- Avoid stain-proof fabrics, carpeting, and Scotchgard spray used for couches and clothing.
- Avoid bedding that is labeled "wrinkle-free," which often means it is made with formaldehyde.

Day 14: Another day to eliminate any toxic products by establishing and committing to new, clean habits. You're almost done, so hang in there!

- Create a no-shoe rule and start removing your shoes at the front door to prevent tracking in chemicals from the street.
- Avoid unnecessary EMF radiation by turning off your WiFi at night. Also, turn your devices to airplane mode when not in use and after you go to bed. Avoid live streaming by downloading programs or games in advance.
- Avoid carrying your cell phone in your front pocket or bra. Avoid Bluetooth earbuds, which emit radiation, and any other wireless devices, like smartwatches or sleep headsets, that use WiFi and can be attached to the body. Keep laptops off your lap and at least one foot from your body.
- Whenever possible, avoid and/or better manage your emotional triggers and the people who create them. I realize this can be challenging, especially if your job or family life is stressful, but setting boundaries with colleagues or loved ones and getting help from trained professionals can help you reduce emotional triggers.
- Avoid synthetic light and use natural light and thick drapes when possible.

- Avoid noise pollution by lowering the volume on radios, televisions, gaming consoles, and computers. Consider adding green plants and wall hangings to help absorb excess noise.
- Discuss with your doctor if your medications are safe, effective, and achieving their goal. Have an end date and/or set a time when dosage can be reduced safely and effectively.

Week Three: Add

It's time to incorporate the good stuff! This week focuses on adding nutrients, clean products, and healing methods to boost your body's detoxification capabilities, while also helping to combat environmental exposures and their toxic effects.

Day 15: It's time to clean up your water. If you can, get a filtration system. No matter how clean you think your well, municipal tap water, or bottled water is, they all have contaminant issues (see chapter 4).

- Add in a water filter that you can afford, preferably one that is reverse osmosis (see page 109). Investigate more options and understand why a water filter is a cost-saving device.
- Replace plastic thermoses, cups, and other reusable beverage containers with glass or stainless-steel options.
- Change to a showerhead with a built-in carbon filter, which removes chlorine. Set a reminder for yourself to buy refills and change the filter every six months.
- Switch to USDA-certified organic coffee and loose-leaf tea (to reduce microplastics found in tea bags). Serve warm beverages in glass or ceramic mugs only, not Styrofoam, plastic, or paper cups (which are often lined with plastic chemicals.)
- Consider switching to a USDA-certified organic brand of beer, wine, or liquor.
- Drink eight to ten glasses of filtered water every day.

Day 16: Add as many nutrient-rich foods to your diet as possible (see chapter 8). For an easy shopping list, see Appendix 1 for the 100 Top Detoxifying Foods to Add to Your Shopping Cart.

- Make a meal plan for one week that includes nutrient-rich, detoxifying foods at every meal and that features at least one high-fiber, detoxifying recipe (see Appendix 4) per day. If any of your meals include fruits or vegetables that are part of the dirty dozen (see page 135), be sure to buy organic versions.
- Replace your cooking oils with cold-pressed organic extra-virgin olive oil to be used when cooking over low heat, and use coconut or MCT oil when cooking at higher temperatures (these have a higher smoke point).
- Replace your most commonly used seasonings with organic spices and herbs, as well as seasoning mixtures, that are sourced and manufactured in the United States.
- Choose free-range chickens raised without antibiotics and/or organic poultry. Select wild-caught fish, particularly the SMASH fish (salmon, mackerel, anchovies, sardines, and herring), which are high in the marine omega-3 fatty acids while also being lower in toxins. Opt for organic grass-fed beef and lean lamb, used in moderation.
- Add in healthy snacks, like mixed nuts, dried fruit without preservatives, fresh fruits, vegetables with hummus or guacamole, and unbuttered, non-GMO homemade popcorn.
- Purchase and use stainless-steel or glass utensils, cups, and plates, and use glass or stainless-steel containers to store food and drink. Also use stainless-steel cooking pans, baking sheets, and food strainers.
- If plastic storage is needed, for safety, use only 100 percent silicone containers, made in the United States. Look for silicone baby bottle nipples with the same characteristics.
- Have a large container with lid and stainless-steel interior handy for picking up takeout food and hot soups.

Day 17: Improve your indoor air quality with the following steps:

- Unless you live in a congested city or directly next to commercial farmland, open the windows each day to allow in fresh, clean air.
- Wet-mop your floors with water only, then dust and vacuum at least once per week to remove dust and the harmful chemicals that cling to it.
- Add indoor plants to help clean the air and support your mental health.
- If you want to scent your home, use only 100 percent essential oils that have been third-party-tested for harmful chemicals.
- Schedule an appointment with a reputable heating, ventilation, and air conditioning (HVAC) service to ensure that you have optimal air filtration and clean vents. Ask if your system is cleaning the air maximally and which MERV (minimum efficiency reporting value) level should be used for greatest air cleaning. (That information is helpful if you need to compare the performance of different filters.) Also, inquire how often the filters need to be cleaned or replaced.
- Add 100 percent cotton, wool, or hemp rugs and carpeting to your home, knowing that they do not off-gas VOC chemicals.
- Consider purchasing a vetted air purifier if you or a member of your household is a smoker, has allergies, and/or has a chronic lung condition like asthma, emphysema, or COPD.
- Use the Recycle Air button in your car (if it has one) when driving through highly trafficked cities or on days with poor air quality.

Day 18: Talk to your healthcare practitioner about adding four "human fertilizer" supplements to your diet. Those four supplements are:

- Omega-3s: 1,000 milligrams combined EPA/DHA daily
- Vitamin D_3: 1,000 to 2,000 IU daily

- Multivitamin: B vitamins, magnesium, selenium, and 150 mcg of iodine (as sodium iodide)
- Probiotic: at least 20 billion CFU daily

Research and purchase the supplements, making sure each one has:

- No preservatives, additives, added colors, added fillers, or added sugars
- Been third-party-tested for quality and purity
- Manufacturer monitoring of product batches for toxic contaminants (lead, cadmium, and mercury); contact the manufacturer if unsure
- An affordable price
- The ability to be taken consistently
- Shown no unusual side effects

See Appendix 5 for online resources on supplement brands and safety.

You can also choose to implement the following steps to simplify your supplement routine:

- Purchase a pill case that can hold a month's supply of pills, which will increase convenience and compliance.
- Use Post-it notes or set alarms on your devices to remind you to take your supplements and get refills when pill counts are low.
- Take your supplements on a full stomach and separate them from medications, if possible, to increase absorption.

Day 19: Time to sweat! Add some physical activity to your day and seek targeted ways to sweat more to increase your blood flow, liver support, and toxin elimination.

- Start by discussing with a healthcare practitioner any limitations you may have for exercise and high-heat activities, like saunas, based on your existing medical conditions and prescription medications.

- Write down all kinds of physical activities you enjoy—or think you might enjoy. Make your list as long as possible and consider nontraditional activities like dance classes, gardening, and rollerblading. (If it moves your body, it counts as exercise.) Then write down when and how you can fit the activities into your daily or weekly routine.
- If you're new to exercise or haven't worked out in a while, start with a routine that's comfortable and pain-free. Aim to do twenty to thirty minutes of aerobic exercise five times per week.
- Wear an extra layer of clothing and a hat for increased sweating, but always make sure to hydrate before, during, and after physical activity.
- Ask your healthcare provider if you are fit for regular use of a sauna and/or steam room. Find a fitness center, YMCA, or other spot with these services and try to go at least three to five times per week.

Day 20: Time to sleep better! Add these targeted ways to sleep better to help your body better eliminate toxins. Use today to consider how to implement the following practices into your daily or weekly routine:

- Keep your bedroom at a cool temperature, preferably between 60°F and 65°F.
- Install dark curtains, blackout shades, or other window coverings to block out as much light as possible.
- Remove computers and other EMF sources from the bedroom.
- Keep an eye mask and earplugs near your bed for times when you want to block out light and noise.
- Consider investing in 100 percent cotton, breathable sheets without formaldehyde to help regulate temperature and reduce toxin exposure.

Day 21: Time to stress less! Add targeted ways to lower your stress, which is another a toxin in the body. Use today to consider how to implement the following practices into your daily or weekly routine:

- Find time to journal, meditate, practice self-reflection, practice breathing exercises, or just be alone with your thoughts.
- Learn to say no to opportunities and events that will add stress or take away from your quality sleep and rest.
- Set time for walks outdoors in green spaces, to leverage the stress-busting healing power of nature.
- Add a regular massage, acupuncture, Reiki, or other form of energy healing, if you have the resources.
- Spend more time with friends and family whom you feel connected to and loved by.
- Mentor others and volunteer for organizations that have a cause in which you believe.
- Consider a form of therapy with a licensed mental health practitioner, many of which are covered by health insurance.
- Plant a flower or vegetable garden to care for.

Beyond Day 22: Allow

Congratulations: You've finished the 21-Day Plan! Give yourself a pat on the back. Detoxifying your refrigerator, pantry, kitchen, bathroom, home, and workspace isn't easy, and making changes to your diet, sleep, exercise, and stress habits takes courage and power.

Retake the Symptom Evaluation Worksheet (pages 282–83) to assess how your symptoms may have improved. Many changes in the plan are long-lasting, so you can expect to see continued results and improvements with no additional effort. If you installed a reverse-osmosis water filter, for example, and replaced some personal-care

Symptom Evaluation Worksheet can help you evaluate whether your symptoms change during and after the 21-Day Plan. To complete the worksheet, rate your symptoms over time on a scale from 1 to 10, 1 being no symptom, 10 being acute symptom. When filling out the Symptom Evaluation Worksheet, keep the following in mind:

- The timing of your symptoms after an exposure occurred
- Intensity of symptoms
- Consistency of symptoms
- Other possible exposures that may contribute to symptoms

Symptom	Day 1	Day 7	Day 14	Day 21	Month 6	Month 9	Month 12	Month 18
Abdominal								
Bloating								
Constipation								
Diarrhea								
Pain								
Abnormal periods								
Frequency								
Heavy flow								
Allergy symptoms								
Itchy eyes								
Runny nose								
Sneezing								
Anxiety								
Blood sugar level (if diabetic)								
Brain fog								
Depression								
Fatigue								
Headache								
Infections								
Respiratory								
Skin/cellulitis								
Urinary tract								

Symptom	Day 1	Day 7	Day 14	Day 21	Month 6	Month 9	Month 12	Month 18
Migraine								
Musculoskeletal symptoms								
Joint pain								
Joint swelling								
Muscle pain								
Muscle weakness								
Shortness of breath								
Skin changes								
Dryness								
Eczema								
Psoriasis								
Rash								
Rosacea								
Tremors								
Weight gain								
Weight loss								

products and home goods with cleaner versions, you'll continue to lower your toxic exposure (as long as you continue to replace the water filter per manufacturer instructions and repurchase clean personal-care and home items when necessary).

Now, it's important to note that change takes time! You didn't develop toxin exposure overnight, and it will take longer than three weeks to effectively lower the amount of toxins in your life. Figuring out the best ways for you personally to eat more nutritious foods, get more exercise, prioritize your sleep, and lower your stress level is going to take some time, and these twenty-one days are the beginning of this experiment, not the end. I hope that the changes you've made in these last three weeks have begun to give you a sense of improvement, but optimal results come when you sustain these habits for years, not weeks.

That's why I suggest focusing on the fourth and final A of the program—Allow. When you finish the 21-Day Plan, allow your new mindset to help make these changes a permanent part of your life. Here are some tips to set that new perspective:

Accept that you can't always be perfect. Our lives are fluid, and there will inevitably be times when you have less access to healthy food, along with less time or money, all of which can influence how easy and convenient it is to lower your exposure. Our living and occupational situations can also change, and the best we can do is to do our best with what we have. Remember that life changes can also reduce stress and help encourage you to do what you can in the moment, when you might be more tempted to give up completely.

Respect the balancing act. There may be times when you have to knowingly expose yourself to toxins. What matters in the long run is that you work to lower your exposure whenever you can. For example, I carry a genetic risk for breast cancer, so I choose to undergo MRIs every few years, even though the screening exposes me to chemicals that could potentially increase risk of health effects.[2] (I also get mammograms every year.) This is an example of the decisions we sometimes must make to balance risk and reward on our health journey.

Create a support system. It's important to have emotional support when you are adopting lifestyle changes. Recruiting a friend or family member can help provide support, as can sharing your journey with those you love, even if they don't participate.

Know that you deserve to be healthy. You are ready and worth it! I've found that, with some patients, they need to be reminded that they deserve to be healthy and feel good.

The 21-Day Plan is a journey that everyone can take, yet everyone's journey will be different. What we all have in common, though, is that everyone—no matter who you are, where you live, what you eat, or what you do—can benefit from a reduction of their toxic exposure while fortifying their body's ability to detoxify. As long as you keep taking steps toward those two goals, no matter how small those steps may be, the rewards will follow, I promise.

APPENDIX 1

100 Top Detoxifying Foods to Add to Your Shopping Cart

ALL THE FOLLOWING foods, in various broad categories, should be purchased USDA-certified organic when available. For certain items, I've listed "organic" here to emphasize the importance of looking for the organic variety.

Fresh Produce

Greens: romaine, Swiss chard, turnip greens, mustard greens, spinach, dandelion greens

Cruciferous vegetables: broccoli, cabbage, cauliflower, kale, bok choy, Brussels sprouts, arugula, radishes

Citrus: oranges, lemons

Tree fruits: pears, apples

Stone fruits: cherries, tangerines, plums, peaches, apricots

Avocados

Carrots

Celery

Grapes: green and red

Melons

Bananas

Small white potatoes (more fiber!)

Sweet potatoes

Artichokes

Tomatoes

Leeks, onions, shallots, chives

Garlic

Mushrooms (washed well and cooked, but particularly button and morels to clear off and deactivate naturally occurring trace carcinogens)[3]

Frozen Produce

Berries: strawberries, cranberries, blueberries, mixed berries, cherries, blackberries, raspberries. Remember to remove produce from its plastic bag or container and switch to glass and stainless steel before heating, microwaving, or storing.

Veggies: broccoli, peas, green beans, corn, zucchini, squash, cauliflower, asparagus, peppers, kale, onions

Beans (including Soy)

Edamame (dry or frozen)

Lentils and beans: garbanzo, black, kidney, pinto

Organic tofu, soy milk, soy crumble, natto (fermented soy)

Dairy and Cheese

Eggs (best if cage-free and omega-3 rich)

Low- or no-sugar flavored or plain Greek yogurt

Milk (2 percent organic cow; almond, soy, oat, hemp, coconut)

Unsalted butter and sour cream (in moderation)

Cheeses (100 percent parmesan, Swiss, mozzarella, ricotta, feta, goat, cottage)

Seafood and Meats

All-white chicken, all-white turkey, 97% low-fat ground chicken or turkey

Wild-caught salmon (fresh or frozen, fished from the Pacific, Canada, or Netherlands)

Shrimp (fresh or frozen, fished from the Pacific, Canada, or Netherlands)

Small fish: mackerel, herring, anchovies, sardines

Naturally smoked salmon or lox (no nitrates or nitrites)

Lean pork filet

Lean ground beef, bison, and/or buffalo (in moderation)

Fresh sliced meats (no nitrites or nitrates added, prioritizing turkey, ham, chicken, roast beef)

Frozen chicken tenders (USDA organic and gluten-free)

Grains, Pasta, and Cereals

Gluten-free grains: millet, amaranth, quinoa, buckwheat, sorghum, cassava, polenta, teff, corn

Whole barley, farro, spelt (if no sensitivities; they contain gluten)

Brown rice

Steel-cut oats (gluten-free) and old-fashioned rolled oats

Pasta (made with USDA organic grains)

Almond- or rice-flour wraps

Pantry Items (preferably sold in glass)

Almond butter (with no fillers like palm oil)

Apple sauce, no added sugar

Dill pickles

Sauerkraut

Olives (all types)

Anchovies

Sardines

Beets

Hearts of palm

Artichokes

Mushrooms

Chicken and vegetable broth (liquid or cubes)

Organic preserves and jams (use with moderation)

Beverages

Loose-leaf tea (all kinds; avoid bagged tea, which can contain microplastics)

Ground or bean coffee (no K-cups)

Sparkling water or seltzer (in glass)

USDA organic wine, beer, spirits

Condiments, Herbs, Spices, Dressings, and Oils

Mustard

No-sugar-added tomato sauce or marinara

Mayonnaise (organic or vegan)

Whole fresh ginger or organic ground

Cinnamon stick or organic Ceylon ground

Chia seeds

Ground flaxseed

Honey (100 percent; otherwise, can contain filler)

Extra-virgin olive oil

Avocado oil

Vinegar (balsamic, distilled white, red wine, apple cider, malt)

Sea salt or Himalayan pink salt

Black pepper

Hot sauce

Chili powder or fresh ground chiles

Curry powder

Fresh or dried herbs and spices, especially turmeric, rosemary, thyme, garlic, sage, basil, oregano, paprika, saffron, nutmeg, cloves, and star anise

Soy sauce (organic)

Raw sugar (100 percent organic)

Maple syrup (pure)

Snack Foods, Desserts, and Treats

Nuts (almonds, walnuts, cashews, Brazil, pistachios, hazelnuts, macadamia)

Seeds (pumpkin, sunflower)

Hummus/chickpea dip

Salsa

Dried fruits (apples, apricots, cranberries, raisins)

Whole-kernel popcorn (pop in brown paper bag)

Potato chips, veggie chips, or pea snaps (cooked in olive or avocado oil only)

Dark chocolate (more than 70 percent cocoa)

Guacamole

Roasted chickpeas

Beef jerky or beef sticks (organic)

Hard-boiled eggs

Kale chips

Baby carrots (with apple butter, hummus, almond butter)

Bone broth

Frozen bananas (with almond butter)

Natural sorbets or ice creams (in moderation)

Dried seaweed (nori)

Rice cakes or pretzels (in moderation)

Granola bars (without added sugar or sweeteners)

Dr. Aly Cohen's Detoxify Food Pyramid

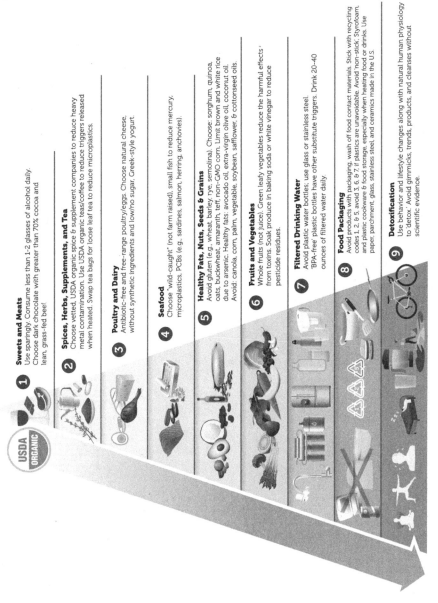

1. Sweets and Meats
Use sparingly. Consume less than 1-2 glasses of alcohol daily. Choose dark chocolate with greater than 70% cocoa and lean, grass-fed beef.

2. Spices, Herbs, Supplements, and Tea
Choose vetted, USDA organic spice & supplement companies to reduce heavy metal contamination. Use USDA organic teas/coffee to reduce triggers released when heated. Swap tea bags for loose leaf tea to reduce microplastics.

3. Poultry and Dairy
Antibiotic-free and free-range poultry/eggs. Choose natural cheese, without synthetic ingredients and low/no sugar, Greek-style yogurt.

4. Seafood
Choose "wild-caught" (not farm raised), small fish to reduce mercury, microplastics, PCBs (e.g. sardines, salmon, herring, anchovies).

5. Healthy Fats, Nuts, Seeds & Grains
Avoid gluten (e.g. wheat, barley, rye, semolina). Choose: sorghum, quinoa, oats, buckwheat, amaranth, teff, non-GMO corn. Limit brown and white rice due to arsenic. Healthy fats: avocado oil, extra-virgin olive oil, coconut oil. Avoid: canola, corn, palm, vegetable, soybean, safflower, & cottonseed oils.

6. Fruits and Vegetables
Whole fruits (not juice). Green leafy vegetables reduce the harmful effects from toxins. Soak produce in baking soda or white vinegar to reduce pesticide residues.

7. Filtered Drinking Water
Avoid plastic water bottles; use glass or stainless steel. 'BPA-free' plastic bottles have other substitute triggers. Drink 20-40 ounces of filtered water daily.

8. Food Packaging
Avoid products with packaging, wash off food contact materials. Stick with recycling codes 1, 2, & 5, avoid 3, 6, & 7; if plastics are unavoidable. Avoid 'non-stick,' Styrofoam, and plastic cookware & food storage, especially when heating food or drinks. Use paper, parchment, glass, stainless steel, and ceramics made in the U.S.

9. Detoxification
Use behavior and lifestyle changes along with natural human physiology to 'detox.' Avoid gimmicks, trends, products, and cleanses without scientific evidence.

APPENDIX 2
Medical and Other Laboratory Testing

I **BELIEVE EVERYONE WITH** access to medical care should get screened for both basic nutrient deficiencies and heavy metals at least once every calendar year. Because both tests are often covered by health insurance, learning your numbers is a low- to no-cost way to know which simple changes you can make to your diet or lifestyle to overhaul your health in real time. If you know you're low in vitamin D, for example, you can take a supplement or consume foods rich in the nutrient—this will boost your nutritional sufficiency and bolster your body's defenses against environmental toxins. The same goes for heavy metals: if you suspect or learn you have been exposed to mercury or cadmium, you can identify and limit your source(s) of exposure while taking targeted steps to help your body better eliminate that chemical. In short, basic nutrient and heavy metal testing takes some of the guesswork out of what to do to improve your health and lower your environmental exposure.

If you have the financial resources, I suggest getting additional lab work, which can give you a more comprehensive snapshot of your nutrient profile and environmental exposure beyond those heavy metals. You may also want to speak with your doctor about getting screened for elevated markers for certain cancers, including colon, breast, and prostate. If you're curious about the water in your home or office, purchase a lab kit to evaluate exactly what's coming out of your tap. And take advantage of free furniture testing for toxic flame retardants.

There's one note about additional testing, though. No test is *necessary* to reduce your environmental exposure, and if you don't have the time or money, invest in the resources you *do* have, such as installing a reverse-osmosis water filtration system in your home and regularly replacing the filter per manufacturer recommendations. Also, you can consume organic, whole foods whenever possible, join a gym or find another way to exercise more frequently, take high-quality brands of my four "human fertilizer" supplements, and prioritize low-toxin personal-care products, cleaning supplies, and other home goods whenever reasonable. Taking these steps will reduce your overall exposure more than any test can.

What's more, it's important to remember that learning your personal data points is beneficial only if you act on the results. Because we're barraged by so many harmful chemicals, making simple changes to reduce your most pervasive toxin exposures will have a significant impact, regardless of testing. At the same time, additional testing can help you make more targeted, personalized, and deliberate changes to your lifestyle to help reduce the exposures that specifically affect you.

Basic Nutritional and Heavy Metal Testing

The easiest way to start the process of basic nutrient and heavy metal testing is to make an appointment with your primary-care doctor, who can order the screenings from a certified national laboratory such as LabCorp or Quest Diagnostics. If you already see or have access to an integrative, functional, or holistic doctor, these practitioners are likely to be more knowledgeable about the nutrient and toxin screenings, as well as how to interpret the results—but it's not necessary to see one of these physicians. Note: While a rheumatologist, endocrinologist, neurologist, and any other medical specialist can also order the tests, some insurance companies require patients to see their primary-care doctor first before agreeing to cover the cost of a visit to a specialized physician.

For best results, you may need to test your nutrient and/or heavy metal levels more than once to evaluate whether any changes made, like reducing certain exposure points or adding dietary supplements, have been effective or if you need to take additional steps or be more aggressive with your new habits.

Insurance companies can be difficult, and even if you call to get answers, there is no guarantee your insurance will pay for the screening. That said, you can up your odds by asking your doctor to include more than one ICD-10 code on your script for a screening. The ICD-10 codes are internationally recognized codes that medical providers submit to insurance companies to justify patient screenings or procedures. Since not all primary-care doctors and specialists are aware of all the ICD-10 codes that can be used to validate these medical screenings, I suggest writing down the following codes associated with each test and asking your doctor if it would be appropriate to include them on your script. You can also look up the ICD-10 codes online at ICD10data.com to find the ones that best correspond with the lab tests you may want to have drawn.

Here are the basic tests, available at national laboratories, that I recommend everyone get:

- *Vitamin deficiencies*: This simple blood test can be ordered to evaluate your levels of vitamin D and B vitamins, in particular B_6, B_{12}, and folate, at a minimum. Possible ICD-10 codes include E56.9, E56, and E61.8.
- *Iodine deficiency*: This simple spot urine test can be ordered to evaluate your iodine levels. Possible ICD-10 codes include E01 and E02; encourage your doctor to use both, as some insurances may not cover the test with one code alone.
- *Heavy metals*: This simple blood test can be ordered to evaluate your levels of arsenic, mercury, cadmium, and lead. Possible ICD-10 codes include T56, T56.894A, T56.894D, and R78.79.

Advanced Nutritional and Heavy Metal Testing

If you have the time and money and want a more comprehensive evaluation of your nutrient levels or chemical exposure, a handful of companies offer blood or urine screenings that can analyze myriad nutrients and chemicals, including the presence or absence of pesticides, plasticizers (phthalates), bisphenol A (BPA), and/or PFAS. Some companies require you to see a licensed practitioner to get tested, while others offer home testing kits that you then send to a lab. Note that these screenings can vary in price and are often not covered by health insurance.

Also, keep in mind that currently there is a limited number of reputable labs offering advanced nutrition and toxin testing, and website information and availability are all subject to change. Finally, some results may be difficult to interpret and may require seeing an integrative or functional medicine practitioner who's knowledgeable in nutrition or toxins for next steps. That said, these tests can help you identify potential problem areas.

Genova NutrEval (https://www.gdx.net/products/nutreval): This test from the company Genova screens for deficiencies and insufficiencies in a range of vitamins, minerals, essential fatty acids, antioxidants, amino acids, and other nutrients. While you will likely have to pay out of pocket for the test—and it's not available in all states—it can be a good option if your primary-care doctor is resistant to basic testing or doesn't have the knowledge to interpret the results, which is true of many physicians trained in conventional Western medicine.

Environmental toxin testing: The following companies offer tests for different environmental toxins. In my opinion, Vibrant provides the most comprehensive screening, but other companies may offer similar analysis. Choose the one that best fits your price range, local availability, and concerns.

Vibrant Labs (www.vibrant-america.com)

Mosaic Diagnostics (www.mosaicdx.com/test/gpl-tox-profile/)

Doctor's Data (www.doctorsdata.com)

Quicksilver Scientific (www.quicksilverscientific.com)

Rupa Health (www.rupahealth.com)

Function Health (www.functionhealth.com)

In addition, some companies offer screenings for specific chemicals. While this is not an exhaustive list, I personally recommend the following companies:

- *Glyphosate exposure testing*: Mosaic Diagnostics (https://mosaicdx.com)
- *Blood perfluoroalkyl (PFAS) testing*: Note that some of the companies listed here operate in only certain regions of the

country. Choose the one that is available in your area and/or works with your price range.

PFAS Exchange (https://pfas-exchange.org/wp-content/uploads/PFAS-Blood-Testing-Document-May-2022.pdf)

EmpowerDx (www.empowerdxlab.com)

Eurofins (www.eurofinsus.com)

NMS Labs (www.nmslabs.com)

SGS Axys Analytical (www.sgsaxys.com)

Quest Diagnostics (www.questdiagnostics.com)

Cancer Screening

For patients with a family history of cancer or any clinical symptoms of the disease—or if you simply want to know as much about your health as possible—speak with your practitioner about getting screened for elevated levels of cancer markers. These screenings, which are exclusive to specific cancers, like liver, ovarian, breast, pancreatic, colon, and prostate, are not diagnostic, meaning they can't tell you or your doctor whether you have the disease. Instead, if a test reveals elevated markers for a certain cancer, you and your physician should make sure you undergo diagnostic testing or have more routine or aggressive diagnostic testing for that cancer.

Since many types of cancers are now affecting younger and younger people, oftentimes before regular diagnostic testing is recommended (e.g., routine mammograms and colonoscopies aren't recommended before age forty-five in people who don't have symptoms or a family history), screening for elevated markers is one way for patients and physicians to catch early stages of the disease. Because cancer is commonly associated with many industrial chemicals, I also believe screening for markers can be advantageous to anyone worried about their environmental exposure. Most screening tests require a simple blood draw or urine sample.

Some health insurances will cover these screening tests, in addition to genetic tests for cancer, which evaluate whether you have inherited any genetic mutations that increase your risk of the disease. To learn which tests may be the most appropriate to determine your personal cancer risk, speak with your primary-care doctor and/or OB-GYN, urologist, gastroenterologist, or other specialist.

The following are the most common cancer markers associated with different types of the disease. If any of these markers come back elevated, discuss with your doctor next steps for evaluation:

- *Liver cancer*, with a test for the marker AFP, ICD-10 codes: C22.0 and C22.8
- *Ovarian cancer*, with a test for the markers CA-125 and HE4, ICD-10 code: Z12.73
- *Breast cancer*, with a test for the marker CA 15-3, ICD-10 code: Z12.39
- *Pancreatic cancer*, with a test for the marker CA 19-9, ICD-10 code: C25.9
- *Colon cancer*, with a test for the marker CEA, ICD-10 code: Z12.11
- *Prostate cancer*, with a test for the markers PSA and free PSA, ICD-10 code: Z12.5

Drinking Water Testing

If you have the resources and are curious to know exactly what's in your water, you can order a home test from the following companies, all which analyze the different types of contaminants that may be coming out of your tap, including lead and PFAS in some instances.

Just remember that tap water contamination can change from season to season, and that testing your home drinking water should never take the place of installing a vetted filtration system, such as reverse osmosis.

- Tap Score (www.mytapscore.com)
- National Testing Laboratories (www.watercheck.com/products/city-check-deluxe)
- Safe Home Test Kits (www.safehometestkits.com/)
- Further resource: www.nytimes.com/wirecutter/reviews/best-water-quality-test-kit-for-your-home/

If money is an issue, skip the home testing and invest in buying the right kind of water filter.

Furniture Testing for Toxic Flame Retardants

As discussed in chapter 7, many sofas, car seats, high chairs, padded chairs, mattresses, and other furniture and home goods are made with materials that contain toxic flame retardants, even if they're labeled organic. If you own any furniture made of polyurethane foam, which has a sponge-like consistency and very small pores, you can send a small sample of the item to Duke University Foam Project (foam.pratt.duke.edu), which will evaluate up to five different samples per household *for free*, mailing you the results in six to eight weeks' time.

APPENDIX 3
DIY Household Cleaners

THE BEST WAY to control the chemicals in your cleaning products is to make your own, which is ridiculously easy to do. All you need to do is buy the ingredients and mix. Most batches last about three months; after that, it's best to toss them, as the natural ingredients start to degrade.

All-Purpose Spray Cleaner

Version A

2 cups boiling water

1 teaspoon liquid castile soap (non-antibacterial, without added fragrance)

½ teaspoon washing soda

Empty spray bottle

Version B

1 cup white vinegar

1 cup warm water

1 tablespoon organic liquid soap

1 teaspoon baking soda

Empty spray bottle

For either version

Combine the ingredients in the spray bottle. Shake well to dissolve the powders. Use to clean nonporous surfaces in your kitchen, bathroom, living room, and bedroom.

Dishwashing Soap

2 cups water

2 tablespoons liquid castile soap (non-antibacterial, without added fragrance)

Empty bottle or large glass jar

1 teaspoon vegetable glycerin

Combine the water and castile soap in the spray bottle. Add the glycerin and stir. Use by applying to a sponge that has been soaked with warm water. If using in an automatic dishwasher, fill only half the soap reservoir to avoid excessive suds.

Oven Cleaner

2 tablespoons castile or nontoxic liquid soap (not detergent)

2 teaspoons borax (inhibits mold growth)

Empty spray bottle

Warm water

Coarse sea salt

Add the soap and borax to the spray bottle and add warm water up to the top. Spray closely to the oven surfaces to avoid inhaling or getting spray in your eyes. Let the solution set for twenty minutes, then scrub with a damp cloth dipped in coarse sea salt. (Or, for tougher spots, scrub with steel wool or a pumice stone, available at most hardware stores.) Once your oven is dry, it's ready for use again.

Note: To pre-treat stains, apply the baking soda first, moisten with water, and let stand overnight. Wipe and rinse.

Mold and Mildew Cleaner

1 cup borax or white vinegar
4 cups water

Empty spray bottle

Combine the borax and water in the spray bottle. Spray on the surface and allow to set before scrubbing or wiping clean; how much you use depends on the severity of the mold or mildew.

Note: To prevent future mold and mildew, limit the sources of moisture in the bathroom by keeping the windows open for at least one hour after showering or whenever damp air invades your home. For serious mold and mildew, consider using a bathroom dehumidifier.

Air Freshener

5 drops of orange, lemon, or lime essential oil (look for 100 percent organic)

2 cups warm water
Empty spray bottle

Combine the essential oil and warm water in the spray bottle. Mist into the air to help diffuse odors. Just be careful not to spray too closely to light-colored or delicate furniture, lest it develops stains.

Stain Remover
For clothing and carpet

¼ cup baking soda or club soda
2 cups warm water

Empty spray bottle

Combine the baking soda and warm water in the spray bottle. Spray on the stain, allow to set for fifteen minutes, then dab with a moist towel to lift the stain.

Glass Cleaner

3 cups water
¼ cup white vinegar
1½ tablespoons lemon juice
Empty spray bottle

Combine the water, vinegar, and lemon juice in the spray bottle. Spray the glass surfaces and wipe clean with a cloth or paper towel.

Wood Polish

1 cup vegetable or olive oil
¼ cup lemon juice
Empty spray bottle

Combine the oil and lemon juice in the spray bottle, making only enough as necessary, as this mixture can go rancid quickly. Spray lightly onto a cloth, then rub into the wood against the grain.

Note: Keep any leftovers refrigerated to prevent spoilage.

Toilet Bowl Cleaner

1 cup borax
3 cups warm water
Empty spray bottle

Combine the borax and warm water in the spray bottle and shake well. Use for cleaning the inside of the bowl.

Note: Clean the seat and rim (where children come into contact with the toilet) with window cleaner, all-purpose cleaner, or equal parts white vinegar and warm water.

Drain Cleaner

½ cup baking soda
½ cup white vinegar
Small jar or bottle
1 quart boiling water

Combine the baking soda and vinegar in the jar and shake well. Pour down the drain and wait fifteen minutes. Carefully pour the boiling water down the drain, dissolving any food, grease, or other materials caught there.

Stainless Steel Polisher

¼ cup baking soda

2 cups water

Quart jar or bottle

Combine the baking soda and water in the jar and shake or stir well. Apply to stainless steel objects using a dry, soft sponge. Allow to sit for fifteen minutes, then wipe off using a moist cloth or sponge.

Laundry Detergent (powdered)

1 bar castile soap, grated

2 cups borax

2 cups washing soda

1 cup baking soda

30 drops essential oil

20-ounce container with airtight lid

Combine the soap, borax, washing soda, baking soda, and essential oil in the container and mix well. Use 1 tablespoon detergent per laundry load.

Note: Close tightly with a lid, especially when storing.

Fabric Softener

½ cup white vinegar

Add the vinegar to the machine at the start of the wash; it will prevent static cling, brighten and soften fabrics, and reduce any strong odor.

APPENDIX 4

Detox Recipes

THE FOLLOWING RECIPES feature foods that boost the body's ability to detoxify, including cruciferous vegetables, alliums (like garlic and onion), and other foods known for their detoxification properties. (For more information on detoxifying foods and what they do in the body, see chapter 8.) Whenever possible, prepare these dishes and drinks using certified-organic ingredients and filtered water, and in cookware, bakeware, and/or with utensils made from glass, high-quality ceramics (not manufactured in China), copper, or stainless steel.

The following recipes are adapted and modified from eatingforyourhealth.org.

Soups

Creamy Cauliflower Soup

Contains fiber, sulforaphane, folate, selenium, and vitamins C and K, among other nutrients.

Makes 8 servings

- 3 tablespoons coconut oil
- 1 teaspoon salt, or to taste
- 3 leeks, trimmed, washed, and thinly sliced
- 2 garlic cloves, roughly chopped
- 1 (2-inch) piece of fresh ginger, peeled and grated
- 1 medium cauliflower, trimmed and roughly cut into chunks
- ½ cup raw Brazil nuts, soaked for at least 2 hours or overnight, drained and rinsed
- 4 cups vegetable or chicken stock
- 1 tablespoon apple cider vinegar or fresh lemon juice
- Hot sauce (optional)

Melt the coconut oil in a large soup pot over medium heat. Add the teaspoon salt and the leeks and sauté for 5 minutes. Add the garlic, ginger, and cauliflower and sauté for another 5 minutes. Add the Brazil nuts and stock, bring to a boil, reduce the heat, cover, and simmer for 30 minutes.

Remove the pot from the heat and let the soup cool for at least 1 hour.

Puree the soup in a high-speed blender until creamy. Season with the vinegar and additional salt to taste. Divide into bowls and serve with hot sauce, if desired.

Pureed Butternut Squash Soup

Contains fiber, selenium, beta carotene, vitamin C, potassium, healthy fats, and organosulfur, among other nutrients.

Makes 10 servings

- 2 tablespoons coconut oil, or as needed
- 1 medium onion, finely chopped
- 1 tablespoon ground cumin
- 1 teaspoon ground cardamom
- ⅛ teaspoon cayenne
- 1 medium butternut squash (about 2½ cups), peeled, seeded, and cubed
- 2 yellow summer squash, diced (or 2 peeled and diced parsnips for a sweeter soup)
- 3 medium carrots, roughly chopped
- 6 cups vegetable stock

Add the coconut oil to a soup pot set over medium heat; add enough oil to coat the bottom of the pot. Add the onion and sauté for 5 minutes, until translucent. Add the spices, stir, and sauté for 1 minute. Stir in the squash and carrots and sauté for another minute. Add the stock, bring to a boil, reduce the heat to low, and simmer for about 15 minutes, until the butternut squash is soft.

Remove the pot from the heat and carefully process (see Note) with an immersion blender until smooth (or transfer to a food processor or blender and puree until smooth, working in batches if necessary). Divide among bowls and serve.

Note: Always use great caution when pureeing hot liquids. If you have time, allow the soup to cool completely before blending. Never fill the container more than half full, and cover the lid with a folded kitchen towel, holding it in place, while you blend the soup.

Barley Miso Soup

Contains fiber, iodine, selenium, and vitamins D_2 and D_3, among other nutrients.

Makes 4 servings

12 cups (3 quarts) filtered water

2 tablespoons tamari or soy sauce (gluten-free if needed)

1 strip of kombu (see Note)

⅓ cup dried shiitake mushrooms, soaked according to package directions

¼ cup dried seaweed (wakame or arame)

¼ block silken tofu, diced

½ cup barley miso, or more as needed (see Note)

Place the water in a large pot and add the tamari and kombu. Bring to a boil over medium-high heat. Add the mushrooms and seaweed, reduce the heat to low, and simmer for about 10 minutes. Add the tofu and turn off the heat.

In a small bowl, mix the miso with about ½ cup of the broth until smooth. Add the miso to the soup and stir well. Do not reheat the soup, but taste before serving, as miso pastes vary in flavor and saltiness; if the broth tastes too thin, stir in more dissolved miso.

Note: Kombu, a type of kelp or seaweed, helps improve the digestibility of beans and legumes. It can be found in some grocery stores, most health food markets, and online. Barley contains gluten, so this miso should not be consumed by anyone who wants to avoid gluten.

Carrot Ginger Soup

Contains beta carotene, organosulfur, healthy fats, antioxidants, folate, magnesium, and fiber, among other nutrients.

Makes 4 servings

- 2 tablespoons coconut oil or extra-virgin olive oil
- 2 medium onions, chopped
- 1½ pounds carrots, peeled and sliced (about 7 medium carrots)
- 1 tablespoon grated fresh ginger
- Salt and black pepper
- 4 cups vegetable stock or filtered water

In a large soup pot, melt the coconut oil over medium heat. Add the onions and sauté for 5 minutes, without browning.

Add the carrots, ginger, and a sprinkling of salt. Cover and cook for 10 minutes. Stir occasionally but do not allow the vegetables to brown.

Add the stock and bring to a boil, reduce the heat to low, cover, and simmer gently for about 15 minutes, until the carrots are tender.

Using an immersion blender, puree the soup in the pot (or transfer to a food processor or blender and process in batches, then return to the pot). Reheat gently, then taste and season with more salt and some pepper.

Quick Gazpacho

Contains fiber, electrolytes, antioxidants, organosulfur, healthy fats, vitamin C, and the antioxidants lutein and zeaxanthin, among other nutrients.

Makes 4 servings

- 1 garlic clove
- 1 tablespoon olive oil
- 2 tablespoons fresh lemon or lime juice (or 1 to 2 tablespoons white vinegar)

1 red bell pepper, cored, seeded, and cut into ½-inch pieces

1 medium cucumber, peeled, seeded, and cut into ½-inch pieces

2 ripe medium tomatoes, cored and cut into ½-inch pieces

1 cup vegetable juice (tomato or other variety you like)

Pinch of sea salt

1 medium red onion, finely chopped (optional)

1 celery stalk, cut into ¼-inch dice (optional)

1 bunch (4 to 8 sprigs) fresh parsley, basil, or cilantro, stems trimmed, leaves roughly chopped (optional)

Hot sauce (optional)

Place the garlic, olive oil, and juice in a food processor and pulse to mince the garlic. Add the bell pepper and cucumber, and pulse several times to chop finely.

Add the tomatoes and vegetable juice and process just to blend; there should still be a bit of chunkiness. Taste and add the salt.

Divide the soup into serving bowls. Garnish with the red onion, celery, and chopped herbs, if desired. Serve with hot sauce on the side, if you like.

Salads

Broccoli Slaw

Contains fiber, folate, sulforaphane, organosulfur, electrolytes, vitamins K and C, probiotics, and the antioxidants lutein and zeaxanthin, among other nutrients.

Makes 12 servings

Slaw

1 large broccoli (about 2 pounds)

1 small red cabbage

1 jícama

½ medium red onion, finely chopped

Dressing

½ cup paleo mayonnaise (made with olive or avocado oil)

2 tablespoons fresh lemon juice

2 tablespoons apple cider vinegar

1 teaspoon salt, or more as needed

Freshly ground black pepper

For serving

1 avocado, peeled and sliced

Make the salad: Separately shred the broccoli, cabbage, and jícama in a food processor using the grating disk. As each grating is finished, transfer the vegetable to a large bowl, then combine the vegetables, stirring well. Add the red onion and stir well.

Make the dressing: In a small bowl, whisk together the mayonnaise, lemon juice, vinegar, 1 teaspoon salt, and a generous quantity of fresh pepper.

Pour the dressing over the broccoli mixture and stir to combine. Taste and add more salt or pepper, if needed.

Allow the salad to sit at room temperature for at least 30 minutes (or 1 hour in the fridge) so the flavors can mingle; you can also leave overnight in the fridge.

Serve the salad with the avocado slices on top.

Apple Bok Choy Salad

Contains fiber, carotenoids, magnesium, sulforaphane, vitamin C, selenium, and probiotics, among other nutrients.

Makes 6 servings

Salad

6 cups finely chopped bok choy (from 1 large head)

1 large apple, cored and shredded or chopped

1 large carrot, shredded or chopped

Dressing

½ cup unsweetened almond, hemp, or soy milk

½ cup raw cashews or Brazil nuts (or ¼ cup raw cashew butter)

¼ cup apple cider vinegar

¼ cup raisins

1 teaspoon Dijon mustard

Make the salad: In a large bowl, combine the bok choy, apple, and carrot.

Make the dressing: Add the almond milk, cashews, vinegar, raisins, and mustard to a food processor or high-powered blender and blend until smooth.

Pour the dressing over salad and toss to combine. Serve.

Dandelion, Jícama, and Orange Prebiotic Salad

Contains fiber, folate, vitamins C, K, and A, dandelion greens, healthy fats, and probiotics, among other nutrients.

Makes 4 servings

1 jícama, diced

½ bunch dandelion greens, trimmed and chopped

3 oranges, peeled, sectioned, and chopped

2 tablespoons extra-virgin olive oil

2 tablespoons balsamic vinegar, or more as desired

Salt and freshly ground black pepper

In a large bowl, combine the jícama, dandelion greens, and oranges. Drizzle with the olive oil and vinegar, and season to taste with salt and pepper. Toss gently and serve.

Lemony Brussels Sprouts Slaw

Contains fiber, sulforaphane, organosulfur, carotenoids, healthy fats, vitamin C, calcium, and potassium, among other nutrients.

Makes 8 servings

Slaw

1½ pounds Brussels sprouts

1 Granny Smith apple

1 daikon radish

1 watermelon radish

4 medium carrots

½ red onion or 1 large shallot

Dressing

2 tablespoons mayonnaise

1 teaspoon Dijon mustard

1 tablespoon grated lemon zest

2 tablespoons fresh lemon juice

¼ cup extra-virgin olive oil

Pinch each of salt and pepper

For serving

fresh finely chopped mint

Make the salad: In a food processor, individually shred the sprouts, apple, radishes, carrots, and red onion. Toss the shredded vegetables in a large bowl and combine well.

Make the dressing: Place the mayonnaise, mustard, lemon zest and juice, olive oil and salt and pepper in a jar with a lid. Cover and shake vigorously.

Dress the slaw, then taste and adjust the seasoning, adding more salt or pepper as desired.

Let the slaw sit in the fridge for about 1 hour, then stir and taste again. Garnish with fresh mint and serve.

Paleo Bok Choy Salad

Contains fiber, selenium, sulforaphane, healthy fats, antioxidants, dandelion greens, vitamin K, and folate, among other nutrients.

Makes 8 servings

8 baby bok choy, cleaned and thinly sliced on the diagonal

8 celery stalks, cleaned and thinly sliced on the diagonal

½ cup olive oil

¼ cup fresh lime juice

1 teaspoon mustard

1 teaspoon grated fresh ginger, or more as needed

1 teaspoon honey

Salt

½ cup toasted Brazil nuts, almonds, walnuts, pumpkin seeds, or dandelion greens

In a large bowl, combine the bok choy and celery.

In a medium bowl, whisk together the olive oil, lime juice, mustard, ginger, honey, and a pinch of salt. Pour over the vegetables and garnish with the nuts, seeds, or dandelion greens. Serve.

Vegetable Side Dishes

Cauliflower Risotto

Contains fiber, sulforaphane, healthy fats, folate, and vitamins A, C, K, and D, among other nutrients.

Makes 8 servings

- 1 medium cauliflower, trimmed and cut into florets
- 1 tablespoon coconut oil
- 1 leek, trimmed, washed, and thinly sliced (white and green parts)
- Sea salt
- 2 garlic cloves, minced
- 2 cups diced seasonal vegetables (asparagus, green peas, sugar snap peas, bell peppers, mushrooms, sun-dried tomatoes; optional)
- 1½ tablespoons tahini
- 1 tablespoon nutritional yeast
- 1 tablespoon miso paste
- 1½ cups vegetable stock
- 1½ cups cooked quinoa, prepared according to package directions
- ½ tablespoon fresh lemon juice
- Black pepper
- 1 bunch fresh parsley, stemmed, leaves roughly chopped

Place the cauliflower florets in the bowl of a food processor and process until the size of rice grains; work in batches, if necessary. Set aside.

Heat the oil in a large skillet over medium heat. Add the leek and a pinch of salt and sauté until softened, about 5 minutes. Add the garlic and sauté a few minutes more, until fragrant. If using the vegetables, add them now in stages, first adding those that take longer to cook, then the more tender others.

When the vegetables (if adding) are tender, add the cauliflower rice.

Separately, whisk together the tahini, yeast, miso paste, and broth in a medium bowl, then add the broth mixture to the skillet and stir well. Add the quinoa and simmer for a few minutes more for the mixture to thicken slightly, but do not overcook.

Remove the risotto from the heat and stir in the lemon juice. Adjust the seasonings with more salt and some pepper. Garnish with the parsley and serve.

Curried Cauliflower

Contains fiber, sulforaphane, healthy fats, electrolytes, organosulfur, vitamin C, curcumin, quercetin, the antioxidants zeaxanthin and lutein, magnesium, selenium, and potassium, among other nutrients.

Makes 4 servings

- 2 tablespoons olive oil, or as needed
- 1 large red onion, finely chopped
- 1 (2-inch) piece fresh ginger, peeled and minced
- 2 garlic cloves, minced
- 1 cauliflower, trimmed and roughly chopped
- 1 (13-ounce can) full-fat coconut milk
- 1 tablespoon curry paste (see Note)
- ¼ teaspoon sea salt

Pour the olive oil into a large sauté pan (with a lid) set over medium heat. Add the red onion and ginger and sauté until softened, about 5 minutes. Add the garlic and continue to cook until fragrant, about 3 more minutes.

Add the cauliflower and sauté another 5 minutes. Stir in the coconut milk, curry paste, and salt. Cover, lower the heat, and simmer for 15 minutes to allow the flavors to blend and the cauliflower to soften. Taste for seasoning, then serve.

Note: Curry paste can be found in the Asian aisle of most supermarkets or online.

Mexican "Rice"

Contains fiber, sulforaphane, organosulfur, the antioxidants lutein and zeaxanthin, healthy fats, potassium, vitamins A and K, and folate, among other nutrients.

Makes 6 servings

- 1 cauliflower, trimmed and chopped
- 1 cup grape tomatoes, quartered
- 4 radishes, trimmed and finely diced
- 1 red bell pepper, cored, seeded, and finely diced

1 bunch fresh cilantro, stemmed leaves finely chopped

1 tablespoon minced onion or scallion white

½ teaspoon ground cumin

Juice of 1 lime (about 2 tablespoons)

1 tablespoon olive oil

Salt

Optional garnishes

1 avocado, peeled and diced

1 jalapeño pepper, seeded and minced

Hot sauce

Place the raw cauliflower in the bowl of a food processor and process until the size of rice grains; work in batches if necessary.

Combine the cauliflower rice, the tomatoes, radishes, bell pepper, cilantro, onion, and cumin in a large bowl. Toss with the lime juice and olive oil. Taste for salt.

Divide into serving portions and, if desired, top with the avocado and garnish with the jalapeño and hot sauce. Serve.

Roasted Brussels Sprouts

Contains fiber, vitamin K, sulforaphane, electrolytes, healthy fats, and folate, among other nutrients.

Makes 4 servings

1 pound Brussels sprouts, washed, trimmed, and halved

½ teaspoon sea salt, or more as needed

1 tablespoon coconut oil or olive oil

1 tablespoon apple cider vinegar

½ teaspoon honey (or 5 drops monk fruit extract)

Preheat the oven to 425°F. Line a baking sheet with parchment paper.

In a medium bowl, toss the Brussels sprouts with the ½ teaspoon salt and the oil. Spread the sprouts evenly on the baking sheet, place in the oven, and roast for 30 minutes, tossing them every 10 minutes or so for even browning.

Season the sprouts with the vinegar, honey, and additional salt to taste. Serve.

Asparagus in Balsamic Butter

Contains fiber, sulforaphane, healthy fats, electrolytes, selenium, choline, and vitamin B_{12}, among other nutrients.

Makes 6 servings

- 3 bunches fresh asparagus, tough bottoms snapped off
- 1 tablespoon extra-virgin olive oil
- Sea salt and black pepper
- 4 tablespoons (½ stick) butter (or olive oil, if avoiding dairy)
- 1 tablespoon tamari
- 1 tablespoon golden balsamic vinegar
- 2 hard-boiled eggs, grated or crumbled

Preheat the oven to 400°F. Line a baking sheet with parchment paper.

Spread the asparagus in a single layer on the baking sheet. Drizzle with the olive oil and sprinkle with some salt and pepper. Bake for 10 to 12 minutes, turning once for even browning, until tender.

In a small saucepan, melt the butter and stir in the tamari and vinegar.

Arrange the roasted asparagus on a serving platter, drizzle with the dressing, and sprinkle with the egg crumbles. Serve.

Main Dishes

Moroccan-Style Chicken Stew

Contains selenium, the antioxidants lutein and zeaxanthin, electrolytes, organosulfur, vitamins C and D, carotenoids, and potassium, among other nutrients.

Makes 8 servings

4 cups chicken stock

1 (6-ounce) can tomato paste

1 teaspoon sea salt, or more as needed

2 teaspoons ground cumin

¼ teaspoon cayenne

⅛ teaspoon ground cinnamon

½ cup raisins

1 large onion, finely chopped

2 tablespoons chopped garlic

2 pounds (3 to 5 medium) sweet potatoes, peeled and cut into small chunks

2 (15-ounce) cans chickpeas, rinsed and drained

3 pounds skinless boneless chicken breasts, cut into small chunks (about 2 cups)

2 cups chopped green vegetables of choice (broccoli, artichoke hearts, zucchini, green beans, etc.)

3 cups cooked rice or millet, warm

In a large soup pot, combine the stock, tomato paste, 1 teaspoon salt, and the spices. Whisk until blended, then add the raisins, onion, garlic, sweet potatoes, chickpeas, and chicken.

Bring to a gentle boil over medium-low heat, then reduce the heat to low, cover, and simmer for 20 minutes.

Add the vegetables and cook another 10 minutes, or until the chicken is no longer pink and the sweet potatoes are soft. Season to taste with more salt, if desired.

Serve the stew over the warm rice or millet.

Breakfast Challenge Turkey Chili

Contains fiber, iron, selenium, folate, healthy fats, electrolytes, sulforaphane, the antioxidants lutein and zeaxanthin, potassium, vitamin C, phosphorus, and choline, among other nutrients.

Makes 6 servings

2 tablespoons olive oil, or enough to coat pan

1½ pounds ground turkey

1 tablespoon chili powder

Sea salt

8 cups chopped high-fiber vegetables (celery, artichoke hearts, cauliflower, mushrooms, kale, zucchini, cabbage, turnips)

2 (15-ounce) cans beans of choice, rinsed and drained (omit for low-carb option)

1 (8-ounce) jar no-added-sugar tomato sauce

1 (8-ounce) jar no-added-sugar salsa

1 to 2 tablespoons apple cider vinegar, or more as needed

1 teaspoon honey (or 6 drops monk fruit extract)

Coat the bottom of a soup pot with the olive oil and heat to shimmering over medium-high heat. Add the ground turkey and break up any clumps, stirring to brown lightly, about 5 minutes.

Add chili powder and 1 teaspoon salt, and sauté for another minute.

Add the vegetables, beans (if using), tomato sauce, and salsa. Stir, reduce the heat to low, and bring to a gentle simmer. Depending on the amount of liquid in the salsa, you may need to add some water or broth to keep the mixture light. Continue to simmer until the liquid mostly evaporates and mixture is the consistency you like, about 20 minutes.

Balance the flavor to your taste with the vinegar, honey, and additional salt to taste. Divide into individual bowls and serve.

Paleo Grass-Fed Beef or Lamb Hash

Contains iron, fiber, folate, selenium, healthy fats, electrolytes, organosulfur, and vitamins A and C, among other nutrients.

Makes 4 servings

2 tablespoons coconut oil, or enough to coat the pan

1 teaspoon sea salt, or more as needed

1 tablespoon curry powder or ras el hanout spice mixture (optional)

1 medium onion, diced

3 garlic cloves, minced

1 red bell pepper, cored, seeded, and diced

1 pound grass-fed ground beef or lamb

4 cups chopped or shredded low-starch veggies (greens, artichoke hearts, cabbage, summer squash, baby spinach)

Water or coconut milk, as needed

Fresh lemon juice

Black pepper

Pour enough oil into a large pot to cover the bottom, then heat to a shimmer over medium-high heat. Add the 1 teaspoon salt and the curry powder (if using) and stir constantly for half a minute—don't let the spices get smoky.

Add the onion, then reduce the heat to medium and cook about 10 minutes, stirring occasionally, until the onion is very soft.

Add the garlic and bell pepper and continue to cook for about 5 minutes, until soft.

Add the meat and stir. Continue to cook, browning the meat for about 10 minutes.

Add the vegetables and a few tablespoons of water or coconut milk, just enough to add some moisture so the vegetables can steam. Cover and cook for 10 to 15 minutes, until the vegetables are soft (adding a bit more water or coconut milk, if necessary, to keep the mixture moist).

Taste and balance the flavor with a little lemon juice, additional salt, and some black pepper. Divide into individual portions and serve.

Pulled Chicken, Squash, and Greens

Contains fiber, selenium, organosulfur, healthy fats, vitamins B_6, B_{12}, and C, choline, and carotenoids, among other nutrients.

Makes 6 servings

2 teaspoons coconut oil

1 teaspoon sea salt, or more as needed

2 large leeks, trimmed, washed, and sliced

¼ cup minced fresh ginger

1 large butternut squash, peeled, seeded, and diced

2 bunches fresh greens, trimmed, leaves and any stems separately chopped (kale, artichoke hearts, collards, chard)

4 cups chicken stock

1 (3-pound) roasted or rotisserie chicken, boned and meat shredded by hand (2 to 3 cups)

Black pepper

1 tablespoon apple cider vinegar

Add the oil and 1 teaspoon salt to a large pot set over medium heat and heat until the oil is shimmering.

Add the leeks and ginger and sauté until they start to color, about 5 minutes. Add the squash and sauté for a couple of minutes, then add the stock and any chopped vegetable stems. Bring to a boil, reduce the heat to low, and simmer for 15 minutes, until the squash is tender.

Add the chopped leaves and shredded chicken, and simmer for an additional 5 minutes. Season with additional salt, some pepper, and a splash of the cider vinegar. Divide into individual portions and serve.

Miso-Crusted Salmon

Contains selenium, omega-3 fatty acids, organosulfur, folate, vitamins C, A, and K, and selenium, among other nutrients.

Makes 6 servings

- 1 large bunch fresh cilantro, trimmed and leaves minced
- 1 bunch scallions (green and white parts), trimmed and minced
- ¾ cup brown or red miso (unpasteurized), or more if needed
- 3 tablespoons grated fresh ginger
- 4 lemons, zested and juiced
- 2 pounds wild-caught salmon fillet, skin removed

Preheat the oven to 375°F. Line a baking sheet with parchment paper.

In a large bowl, combine the cilantro, scallions, miso paste, ginger, lemon zest, and 2 tablespoons of the lemon juice. Stir to make a thick paste.

Place the salmon fillet on the baking sheet and spread the top with a thick layer of the paste. Bake for 20 to 25 minutes, checking for doneness.

Let the salmon rest for a few minutes, then cut into 6 portions and serve.

Desserts and Treats

Blueberry Chia Seed Pudding

Contains fiber, antioxidants, vitamin C, selenium, potassium, and calcium, among other nutrients.

Makes 10 servings

- 2 cups vanilla almond milk
- ¾ cup fresh or frozen blueberries, plus 1 cup fresh berries for garnish
- ½ cup chia seeds
- 1 teaspoon ground cinnamon
- ½ teaspoon almond extract
- 2 tablespoons honey (or 16 drops monk fruit extract)
- ¼ cup crushed Brazil nuts, for garnish

In a food processor, combine the almond milk and ¾ cup of blueberries, processing until smooth.

Pour the blueberry puree into a large bowl and add the chia seeds, cinnamon, almond extract, and honey. Cover and refrigerate (stirring occasionally) for at least 2 hours and up to 24 hours.

To serve, portion into serving bowls and garnish with the fresh berries and the Brazil nuts.

Gluten-Free Banana Bread

Contains fiber, potassium, choline, vitamin B_{12}, selenium, and magnesium, among other nutrients.

Makes 1 loaf (8 to 10 servings)

- 3 very ripe bananas
- 1 cup almond butter
- 2 large eggs
- ¼ cup honey (optional)
- 1 cup almond meal
- 1 teaspoon baking soda
- 1 teaspoon baking powder
- ¼ teaspoon sea salt
- ¼ cup chocolate chips (optional)

Preheat the oven to 350°F. Line a 9 by 5-inch loaf pan with parchment paper.

In a large bowl, mash the bananas, then add the almond butter, eggs, and honey (if using). Mix well, then add the almond meal, baking soda, baking powder, and salt. Stir until just blended, then fold in the chocolate chips.

Pour the batter into the loaf pan and bake for 60 minutes, or until dry in the middle.

Ginger Lemon Truffles

Contains fiber, selenium, healthy fats, folate, vitamins C and E, zinc, iron, and magnesium, among other nutrients.

Makes 60 truffles

- 1 (6-inch) piece fresh ginger, grated with Microplane
- 1 pound desiccated coconut
- 5 lemons, zested and juiced
- ¼ cup pure maple syrup (or honey, stevia, monk fruit extract, etc.)
- 1 teaspoon alcohol-free vanilla extract
- 1 (16-ounce) jar organic cashew butter
- ¼ cup ground Brazil nuts
- ¼ teaspoon sea salt
- 1½ cups hulled hemp seeds

In a large bowl and either using a kitchen mixer or by hand with a whisk, combine all the ingredients except the hemp seeds until well mixed. Taste and adjust, adding additional ingredients as desired.

Using a 1-ounce cookie scoop, scoop out portions of the mixture and roll into little balls with gloved hands.

Place the hemp seeds in a shallow dish. Drop the balls into the dish one at a time, rolling them around in the seeds to coat well.

Place the truffles on a platter and chill until ready to serve. (Note: The truffles will keep for one week.)

Avocado and Berry Ice Cream

Contains fiber, healthy fats, vitamin C, and electrolytes, among other nutrients.

Makes 4 servings

1 ripe Haas avocado, peeled

2 ripe bananas, peeled

1 cup frozen blackberries or other berries (from 12-ounce bag)

Pinch of sea salt

1 teaspoon lemon juice, or as needed

½ (13-ounce) can full-fat coconut milk

Cut the avocado and bananas into 1-inch pieces and place on a small sheet or plate. Place in the freezer for 2 to 3 hours.

Place the frozen avocado and banana pieces with the remaining ingredients in a blender or food processor, and process until smooth, adding a little water as needed to obtain the desired consistency. Serve immediately.

Fudgy Maple–Black Bean Brownies

Contains fiber, iron, choline, B_{12}, selenium, healthy fats, and electrolytes, among other nutrients.

Makes 16 brownies

⅓ cup coconut oil or butter, melted, plus more for greasing pan

1 (15-ounce) can black beans, drained and rinsed

3 large eggs

¼ cup raw cacao powder

⅛ teaspoon sea salt

1 teaspoon alcohol-free vanilla extract

¼ cup pure maple syrup

⅓ cup gluten-free chocolate chips or chunks

⅓ cup chopped raw Brazil nuts

Preheat the oven to 350°F. Grease an 8-inch square baking pan with some coconut oil.

Place the beans, eggs, ⅓ cup coconut oil, the cacao powder, salt, vanilla, and maple syrup in a food processor and blend until smooth. Remove the blade and gently stir in the chocolate chips and Brazil nuts.

Transfer the mixture to the baking pan and smooth the top. Bake for 35 minutes, or until the brownies are set in the center and a toothpick comes out clean.

Remove the pan from the oven and let the brownies cool. Cut into 9 squares (3 by 3 cuts). Note: These are best served warm.

Beverages

Dr. Cohen's Nontoxic Electrolyte Supplement Drink

Contains all the electrolytes, magnesium, potassium, sodium, chloride, and calcium.

Makes 2 to 3 servings

½ cup of your favorite juice (without added synthetic sweeteners, preferably bought in a glass bottle)

2 cups filtered water

2 pinches Himalayan pink salt or sea salt

Place the juice, water, and salt in a 20-ounce glass or stainless-steel water bottle and stir well. Chill until ready to serve. (Note: The drink should stay fresh for about seven days when kept refrigerated.)

Super Simple Smoothie

Contains healthy fats, fiber, vitamin C, and potassium, among other nutrients.

Makes 2 servings

½ ripe avocado

1 cup organic strawberries, washed and hulled

1 ripe banana

2 cups almond or coconut milk

Place the avocado, strawberries, banana, and almond milk in a blender. Blend until smooth, then enjoy.

Green Detox Smoothie

Contains fiber, folate, curcumin, calcium, potassium, and healthy fats, among other nutrients.

Makes 2 servings

- 1 cup frozen berries of choice
- 2 cups baby spinach leaves
- ½ teaspoon ground cinnamon
- ¼ teaspoon ground turmeric
- 1 tablespoon unsweetened cocoa powder
- ¼ teaspoon cayenne (optional)
- ¼ cup full-fat coconut milk
- 1 cup unsweetened green tea (iced or room temperature), or more as needed

Place all the ingredients in a high-speed blender and blend until pureed. Enjoy.

Cinnamon Warming Tea

Contains potassium and calcium, among other nutrients.

Makes 8 servings

- 2 quarts filtered water
- 8 cinnamon sticks
- 2 bags of green tea
- Honey, for serving

Bring the water and cinnamon sticks to a boil in a medium pot over high heat. Reduce the heat to low and simmer for 20 to 30 minutes. Pour the tea into a tea pot with the tea bags and steep for 10 minutes. Serve with local raw honey for added antimicrobial benefits and sweetness.

Golden Milk

Contains healthy fats, curcumin, vitamin C, calcium, and potassium, among other nutrients.

Makes 4 servings

- 1 (13-ounce) can full-fat coconut milk
- 1 cup filtered water
- 2 tablespoons turmeric powder (or 4-inch piece turmeric root, grated)

- 2 tablespoons honey (or 16 drops monk fruit extract)
- 1 (2-inch) piece fresh ginger, grated
- 2 cinnamon sticks
- 5 black peppercorns

Combine all the ingredients in a saucepan set over medium heat. Simmer for 20 minutes, then strain through a fine-mesh strainer or cheesecloth into individual mugs. Serve hot.

APPENDIX 5
Online Resources

Toxic chemical overviews and information

Agency for Toxic Substances and Disease Registry: www.atsdr.cdc.gov/index.html

Collaborative for Health and Environment Toxicant and Disease Database: www.healthandenvironment.org/our-work/toxicant-and-disease-database/?showdisease=699

Environmental Health News: www.ehn.org

Healthy Environment and Endocrine Disruptor Strategies (HEEDS): www.heeds.org

Environmental Working Group: www.ewg.org

Program on Reproductive Health and the Environment: www.prhe.ucsf.edu

Women's Voices for the Earth: www.womensvoices.org

Icahn/Mount Sinai Environmental Health: www.icahn.mssm.edu/research/pehsu/information

Personal-care products and cosmetics

Environmental Working Group Skin Deep Database: www.ewg.org/skindeep

Apps: Healthy Living, Yuka, Clearya, Think Dirty

Cleaning/household products

Environmental Working Group: www.ewg.org

Consumer Product Information Database (CPID): www.whatsinproducts.com

Flame-retardant and PFAS-free products

Green Science Policy: www.greensciencepolicy.org

PFAS Central: www.pfascentral.org

Mattress/furniture testing for flame retardants

Duke University Foam Project: foam.pratt.duke.edu

Food packaging/food contact information

Food Packaging Forum: www.foodpackagingforum.org

Drinking water filtration

Environmental Protection Agency (EPA): www.epa.gov/ground-water-and-drinking-water/national-primary-drinking-water-regulations

Centers for Disease Control and Prevention: www.cdc.gov/healthywater/drinking/home-water-treatment/water-filters/step3.html

Natural Resources Defense Council: www.nrdc.org/stories/whats-your-drinking-water

Environmental Working Group: www.ewg.org/tapwater/water-filter-guide.php

Drinking water quality ratings by zip code

Environmental Working Group: www.ewg.org/tapwater/

Drinking water testing

Tap Score: www.mytapscore.com

National Testing Laboratories: www.watercheck.com/products/city-check-deluxe

Safe Home Test Kits: www.safehometestkits.com/

Further resource: www.nytimes.com/wirecutter/reviews/best-water-quality-test-kit-for-your-home/

Furniture and textiles

Global Organic Textile Standard (GOTS): www.global-standard.org

Green Science Policy: www.greensciencepolicy.org

Building materials
Green Seal: www.greenseal.org/splash/
HPD Collaborative: www.hpd-collaborative.org
Habitable: www.habitablefuture.org
International Living Future Institute: www.living-future.org/lpc/
Cradle to Cradle Products Innovation Institute: www.c2ccertified.org

Gardening/farming and pesticides
Beyond Pesticides: www.beyondpesticides.org
Organic Farmers Association: www.organicfarmersassociation.org
US Environmental Protection Agency: www.epa.gov/safepestcontrol/integrated-pest-management-ipm-principles

EMF, WiFi, and microwave radiation
Environmental Health Trust: www.ehtrust.org
The BabySafe Project: www.babysafeproject.org
Phone Gate: www.phonegatealert.org

Supplement Information

Quality/purity
ConsumerLab: www.consumerlab.com
Labdoor: www.labdoor.com

Safety/drug interactions
Memorial Sloane Kettering About Herbs Database: www.mskcc.org/cancer-care/diagnosis-treatment/symptom-management/integrative-medicine/herbs/search
Department of Defense Dietary Supplement Resource-Operation Supplement Safety: www.opss.org/disclaimer

Natural Medicines Database (NatMed): www.naturalmedicines.therapeuticresearch.com

NIH Dietary Supplement Label Database: www.ods.od.nih.gov/Research/Dietary_Supplement_Label_Database.aspx

NIH Office of Dietary Supplements: www.ods.od.nih.gov

Acknowledgments

This book was brought to life by many people and pets. I'll begin with my dog Truxtun, whose illness set me on a path toward understanding environmental health. Without his environmental story, there would not be my own story; Oliver and Charlie, my rescue cat and dog, who remain steadfast supporters of my company and never cease to pour unconditional love and affection on me daily, especially during the stressful periods while writing this book.

My patients who keep me grounded, fill me with purpose, and allow me to practice the kind of medicine that makes me proud. It is a privilege to join you on your journey of healing.

My friends (too many to mention and I don't want to forget anyone, or I'll be in the doghouse!), thank you for listening to me . . . the power of this cannot be underestimated nor underappreciated.

Thank you to my mentors and colleagues in environmental health awareness, advocacy, and education: Johanna Congleton, Heather White, Devra Davis, and Ken Cook. Also, organizations such as Cancer Schmancer, Environmental Health News (EHN), Environmental Working Group (EWG), Collaborative for Health and Environment (CHE), Environmental Health Trust (EHT), Healthy Environment and

Endocrine Disruptor Strategies (HEEDS), and Women's Voices for the Earth (WVE); they all play a critical role in moving environmental health awareness forward, and I appreciate your support over the years.

My colleagues in the "Health and Wellness" village who have reached out a hand to lift me up; David Perlmutter, Amy Hebert, Dhru Purohit, Mona Sharma, William Li, Mark Hyman, Terry Wahls, Chase Chewning, Susan Holland and Fran Drescher, Robert Lustig, Felice Gersh, Ronald Hoffman, Darshan Shah, Max Lugavere, Ashley Koff, and Madiha Saeed.

I have had the great privilege of learning from some of the foremost scientists and physicians in the world, and I am grateful for their unparalleled instruction and generosity with their knowledge. These mentors include Integrative Medicine pioneers Andrew Weil and colleagues in the endocrine-disrupting chemical (EDC) research world, Chris Kassotis, Pete Myers, Jane Munke, Shanna Swan, Maricel Maffini, Jerry Heindel, and Christopher Weis, among many others. I would like to especially thank my co-author for two previous texts, Frederick vom Saal, who has been a friend and champion of my efforts to get this information into all educational arenas, especially high school curricula. His support and guidance represent the purist definition of a true mentor.

I'd like to thank my physician colleagues who have rallied behind me and walked beside me on the road of integrative medicine, including Mikhail Kogan, Vivian Kominos, Maria Benito, Marie Steinmetz, Suzanne Bartlett Hackenmiller, Victoria Maizes, and SiriChand Khalsa.

A big thank you to Tieraona Low Dog, MD, who continues to share her immeasurable wisdom with me and has shepherded my environmental health curricula into three integrative medicine physician-training programs.

I want to thank those most responsible for actualizing this book and bringing it into the light; Bonnie Solow for your unwavering support and championing my mission from the start; Sarah Toland for your gift of language and gently guiding me through the emotional process of putting thoughts into written form; Kyle Czepiel for your beautiful graphic design work; Ronnie Alvarado, Leah Miller, Maria Espinosa, Lily Soroka, and the entire team at Simon & Schuster—your knowledge, guidance, and patience have been remarkable.

And finally, I want to express my deepest love and gratitude for my family, especially my amazing parents and big brother, who have been faithfully by my side and cheering me on throughout the longest stretch of my life's journey. To my two magnificent sons, whose endless humor, love, sarcasm, sweetness, understanding (and did I mention sarcasm?) allowed me to "juggle many balls in the air" during a busy and exciting time in their lives. Lastly, I'd like to thank my husband, Stephen Lewis, MD, who has acted often as my therapist, medical consultant, lawyer, and best friend for over two decades, and without a doubt during the last few years writing this book. Your humor and love keep me going.

Notes

Introduction

1. Ian Urbina, "Think Those Chemicals Have Been Tested?" *New York Times*, April 13, 2013, https://www.nytimes.com/2013/04/14/sunday-review/think-those-chemicals-have-been-tested.html.
2. Aly Cohen and Frederick vom Saal, *Non-Toxic: Guide to Living Healthy in a Chemical World* (Oxford, UK: Oxford University Press, 2020).

Chapter 1: The Smoking Gun: Environmental Chemicals

1. Christopher D. Kassotis et al., "Endocrine-Disrupting Chemicals: Economic, Regulatory, and Policy Implications," *Lancet Diabetes & Endocrinology* 8, no. 8 (August 2020): 719–30, https://doi.org/10.1016/S2213-8587(20)30128-5.
2. Aly Cohen and Frederick vom Saal, *Non-Toxic: Guide to Living Healthy in a Chemical World* (Oxford, UK: Oxford University Press, 2020).
3. Ian Urbina, "Think Those Chemicals Have Been Tested?" *New York Times*, April 13, 2013, https://www.nytimes.com/2013/04/14/sunday-review/think-those-chemicals-have-been-tested.html.
4. American Pregnancy Association, "Foods to Avoid During Pregnancy," https://americanpregnancy.org/healthy-pregnancy/pregnancy-health-wellness/foods-to-avoid-during-pregnancy/.
5. Lisa Frack and Becky Sutton, "3,163 Ingredients Hide Behind the Word 'Fragrance,'" Environmental Working Group, February 2, 2010, https://www.ewg.org/news-insights/news/3163-ingredients-hide-behind-word-fragrance.
6. Yufei Wang and Haifeng Qian, "Phthalates and Their Impacts on Human Health," *Healthcare* 9, no. 5 (May 2021): 603, https://doi.org/10.3390/healthcare9050603.
7. Shanaz H. Dairkee et al., "Reduction of Daily-Use Parabens and Phthalates Reverses Accumulation of Cancer-Associated Phenotypes within Disease-Free Breast Tissue of Study Subjects," *Chemosphere* 322 (May 2023), https://doi.org/10.1016/j.chemosphere.2023.138014.
8. Maria Gloria Luciani-Torres et al., "Exposure to the Polyester PET Precursor—Terephthalic Acid Induces and Perpetuates DNA Damage-Harboring Non-Malignant Human Breast Cells," *Carcinogenesis* 36, no. 1 (January 2015): 168–76, https://doi.org/10.1093/carcin/bgu234.
9. Stephen M. Rappaport and Martyn T. Smith, "Environment and Disease Risks,"

Science 330, no. 6003 (October 2010): 460–61, https://www.science.org/doi/10.1126/science.1192603.
10. Leonie Elizabeth et al., "Ultra-Processed Foods and Health Outcomes: A Narrative Review," *Nutrients* 12, no. 7 (June 2020): 1,955, https://doi.org/10.3390/nu12071955.
11. World Health Organization, "An Estimated 12.6 Million Deaths Each Year Are Attributable to Unhealthy Environments," March 15, 2016, https://www.unep.org/news-and-stories/story/estimated-126-million-deaths-each-year-are-attributable-unhealthy.
12. National Council on Aging, "Chronic vs. Acute Medical Conditions: What's the Difference?" February 15, 2024, https://www.ncoa.org/article/chronic-versus-acute-disease.
13. Endocrine Science Matters, "Non-Monotonic Dose Responses," https://endocrinesciencematters.org/non-monotonic-dose-responses-2/non-monotonic-dose-responses-technical-overview/.
14. Ibid.
15. Stephen J. Genuis et al., "Human Excretion of Bisphenol A: Blood, Urine, and Sweat (BUS) Study," *Journal of Environmental Public Health* 2012, no. 1 (December 2011), https://doi.org/10.1155/2012/185731.
16. State of Washington Department of Ecology, "Phthalates," https://ecology.wa.gov/waste-toxics/reducing-toxic-chemicals/addressing-priority-toxic-chemicals/phthalates.
17. Andrea Baccarelli and Valentina Bollati, "Epigenetics and Environmental Chemicals," *Current Opinion in Pediatrics* 21, no. 2 (April 2009): 243–51, https://doi.org/10.1097%2Fmop.0b013e32832925cc.
18. Monish Darda, "Four Pillars of a Consequential and Enduring Company," *Forbes*, March 17, 2023, https://www.forbes.com/sites/forbestechcouncil/2023/03/17/four-pillars-of-a-consequential-and-enduring-company.
19. Endocrine Society, "Endocrine-Disrupting Chemicals (EDCs)," January 24, 2022, https://www.endocrine.org/patient-engagement/endocrine-library/edcs.
20. Cohen and vom Saal, *Non-Toxic*.
21. Endocrine Society, "Endocrine-Disrupting Chemicals (EDCs)."
22. World Health Organization, "State of the Science of Endocrine Disrupting Chemicals 2012," June 6, 2012, https://www.who.int/publications/i/item/9789241505031.
23. David Furman et al., "Chronic Inflammation in the Etiology of Disease across the Life Span," *Nature Medicine* 25, no. 12 (December 2019): 1,822–32, https://doi.org/10.1038/s41591-019-0675-0.
24. Ibid.
25. Cleveland Clinic, "Inflammation," https://my.clevelandclinic.org/health/symptoms/21660-inflammation.
26. Mihai G. Netea et al., "Innate and Adaptive Immune Memory: An Evolutionary Continuum in the Host's Response to Pathogens," *Cell Host & Microbe* 25, no. 1 (January 2019): 13–26, https://doi.org/10.1016/j.chom.2018.12.006.
27. Cleveland Clinic, "Coronaviruses Have Been Around for Centuries: What Differentiates COVID-19?" March 4, 2020, https://consultqd.clevelandclinic.org/coronaviruses-have-been-around-for-centuries-what-differentiates-2019-ncov.
28. Chang-Hung Kuo et al., "Immunomodulatory Effects of Environmental Endocrine Disrupting Chemicals," *Kaohsiung Journal of Medical Sciences* 28, no. 7 (2012): S37–S42, https://www.sciencedirect.com/science/article/pii/S1607551X12001556.

29. Hans-Joachim Lehmler et al., "Exposure to Bisphenol A, Bisphenol F, and Bisphenol S in U.S. Adults and Children: The National Health and Nutrition Examination Survey 2013–2014," *ACS Omega* 3, no. 6 (June 2018): 6,523–32.
30. Carolyn Beans, "How 'Forever Chemicals' Might Impair the Immune System," *Proceedings of the National Academy of Sciences of the United States of America* 118, no. 15 (April 2021), https://www.pnas.org/doi/10.1073/pnas.2105018118.
31. National Institute of Environmental Health Sciences, "Perfluoroalkyl and Polyfluoroalkyl Substances (PFAS)," https://www.niehs.nih.gov/health/topics/agents/pfc/index.cfm.

Chapter 2: Your Body on Chemicals

1. Laura Vargas-Parada, "Research Round-Up: Autoimmune Disease," *Nature*, July 14, 2021, https://www.nature.com/articles/d41586-021-01834-x.
2. Fariha Angum et al., "The Prevalence of Autoimmune Disorders in Women: A Narrative Review," *Cureus* 12, no. 5 (May 2020): e8094, https://www.cureus.com/articles/31952-the-prevalence-of-autoimmune-disorders-in-women-a-narrative-review.
3. Lucy McDonnell et al., "Association between Antibiotics and Gut Microbiome Dysbiosis in Children: Systematic Review and Meta-Analysis," *Gut Microbes* 13, no.1 (2021), https://www.tandfonline.com/doi/full/10.1080/19490976.2020.1870402.
4. Clean Label Project, "Protein Powder," https://cleanlabelproject.org/protein-powder-white-paper/.
5. Center for Consumer Freedom, "5 Chemicals Lurking in Plant-Based Meats," July 17, 2021, https://consumerfreedom.com/2021/07/5-chemicals-lurking-in-plant-based-meats/.
6. Samara Geller, "BPA Update: Tracking the Canned Food Phaseout," Environmental Working Group, November 2, 2020, https://www.ewg.org/news-insights/news/bpa-update-tracking-canned-food-phaseout.
7. Cleveland Clinic, "Dysbiosis," https://my.clevelandclinic.org/health/diseases/dysbiosis.
8. Huihui Xu et al., "The Dynamic Interplay between the Gut Microbiota and Autoimmune Diseases," *Journal of Immunology Research* 2019, no. 1 (October 2019), https://www.ncbi.nlm.nih.gov/pmc/articles/PMC6854958/.
9. Tomas Hrncir, "Gut Microbiota Dysbiosis: Triggers, Consequences, Diagnostic and Therapeutic Options," *Microorganisms* 10, no. 3 (March 2022): 578, https://doi.org/10.3390/microorganisms10030578.
10. Angum et al., "The Prevalence of Autoimmune Disorders in Women."
11. Maurizio Cutolo and Rainer H. Straub, "Sex Steroids and Autoimmune Rheumatic Diseases: State of the Art," *Nature Reviews Rheumatology* 16, no. 11 (November 2020): 628–24, https://pubmed.ncbi.nlm.nih.gov/33009519/.
12. Ibid.
13. Diana R. Dou et al., "Xist Ribonucleoproteins Promote Female Sex-Biased Autoimmunity," *Cell* 187, no. 3 (February 2024): P733–49.e16, https://www.cell.com/cell/fulltext/S0092-8674(24)00002-3.
14. Michael Edwards, Rujuan Dai, and S. Ansar Ahmed, "Our Environment Shapes Us: The Importance of Environment and Sex Differences in Regulation of Autoantibody Production," *Frontiers in Immunology* 9, no. 478 (March 2018),

https://www.frontiersin.org/journals/immunology/articles/10.3389/fimmu.2018.00478/full.

15. A. Nicholson et al., *The Convergence of Infectious Diseases and Noncommunicable Diseases: Proceedings of a Workshop* (Washington, DC: National Academies Press, 2019).

16. Sandrine P. Claus, Herve Guillou, and Sandrine Ellero-Simatos, "The Gut Microbiota: A Major Player in the Toxicity of Environmental Pollutants?" *NPJ Biofilms and Microbiomes* 2, no. 16,003 (May 2016), https://doi.org/10.1038%2Fnpjbiofilms.2016.3.

17. Elizabeth Thursby and Nathalie Juge, "Introduction to the Human Gut Microbiota," *Biochemical Journal* 474, no. 11 (May 2017): 1,823–36, https://doi.org/10.1042%2FBCJ20160510.

18. Yi Mou et al., "Gut Microbiota Interact with the Brain through Systemic Chronic Inflammation: Implications on Neuroinflammation, Neurodegeneration, and Aging," *Frontiers in Immunology* 13 (April 2022), https://doi.org/10.3389/fimmu.2022.796288.

19. Ji Youn Yoo et al., "Gut Microbiota and Immune System Interactions," *Microorganisms* 8, no. 10 (October 2020): 1,587, https://doi.org/10.3390/microorganisms8101587.

20. Selma P. Wiertsema et al., "The Interplay between the Gut Microbiome and the Immune System in the Context of Infectious Diseases throughout Life and the Role of Nutrition in Optimizing Treatment Strategies," *Nutrients* 13, no. 2 (March 2021): 886, https://doi.org/10.3390/nu13030886.

21. Walaa K. Mousa, Fadia Chehadeh, and Shannon Husband, "Microbial Dysbiosis in the Gut Drives Systemic Autoimmune Diseases," *Frontiers in Immunology* 13, no. 906,258 (October 2022), https://doi.org/10.3389%2Ffimmu.2022.906258.

22. Claus, Guillou, and Ellero-Simatos, "The Gut Microbiota."

23. Ian Rowland et al., "Gut Microbiota Functions: Metabolism of Nutrients and Other Food Components," *European Journal of Nutrition* 57, no. 1 (April 2017): 1–24, https://doi.org/10.1007%2Fs00394-017-1445-8.

24. "Study Shows How Serotonin and a Popular Anti-Depressant Affect the Gut's Microbiota," *Science Daily*, September 6, 2019, https://www.sciencedaily.com/releases/2019/09/190906092809.htm.

25. Hrncir, "Gut Microbiota Dysbiosis."

26. Ibid.

27. Pengcheng Tu et al., "Gut Microbiome Toxicity: Connecting the Environment and Gut Microbiome-Associated Diseases," *Toxics* 8, no.1 (March 2020): 19, https://doi.org/10.3390%2Ftoxics8010019.

28. Stephen M. Rappaport and Martyn T. Smith, "Environment and Disease Risks," *Science* 330, no. 6003 (October 2010): 460–61, https://doi.org/10.1126%2Fscience.1192603.

29. Nicole Mohajer et al., "Obesogens: How They Are Identified and Molecular Mechanisms Underlying Their Action," *Frontiers in Endocrinology* 12 (November 2021): 780888, https://doi.org/10.3389/fendo.2021.780888.

30. Jerrold J. Heindel et al., "Obesity II: Establishing Causal Links Between Chemical Exposures and Obesity," *Biochemical Pharmacology* 199 (May 2022): 115015, http://dx.doi.org/10.1016/j.bcp.2022.115015.

31. Mohajer et al., "Obesogens."

32. Lydia Lynch et al., "iNKT Cells Induce FGF21 for Thermogenesis and Are Required for Maximal Weight Loss in GLP1 Therapy," *Cell Metabolism* 24, no. 3 (September 2016): 510–19, https://doi.org/10.1016/j.cmet.2016.08.003.

33. Heindel et al., "Obesity II."
34. Ibid.
35. Ibid.
36. Iva Kladnicka et al., "Obsogens in Foods," *Biomolecules* 12, no. 5 (May 2022): 680, https://doi.org/10.3390%2Fbiom12050680.
37. Heindel et al., "Obesity II."
38. Ibid.
39. Ibid.
40. Green Science Policy Institute, "Bisphenols & Phthalates: Are They Disrupting Our Hormones?" https://greensciencepolicy.org/harmful-chemicals/bisphenols-phthalates/.
41. Heindel et al., "Obesity II."
42. Kladnicka et al., "Obsogens in Foods."
43. Ibid.
44. Jerrold J. Heindel and Bruce Blumberg, "Environmental Obesogens: Mechanisms and Controversies," *Annual Review of Pharmacology and Toxicology* 59 (January 2016): 89–106, https://doi.org/10.1146%2Fannurev-pharmtox-010818-021304.
45. Heindel et al., "Obesity II."
46. Environmental Working Group, "Perfluorooctanoic Acid (PFOA)," 2021, https://www.ewg.org/tapwater/contaminant.php?contamcode=E207.
47. Alissa Cordner et al. "Guideline Levels for PFOA and PFOS in Drinking Water: The Role of Scientific Uncertainty, Risk Assessment Decisions, and Social Factors," *Journal of Exposure Science & Environmental Epidemiology* 29, no. 2 (2019): 157–71, https://doi.org/10.1038/s41370-018-0099-9.
48. World Health Organization, "IARC Monographs Evaluate the Carcinogenicity of Perfluorooctanoic Acid (PFOA) and Perfluorooctanesulfonic Acid (PFOS)," December 1, 2023, https://www.iarc.who.int/news-events/iarc-monographs-evaluate-the-carcinogenicity-of-perfluorooctanoic-acid-pfoa-and-perfluorooctanesulfonic-acid-pfos/.
49. Heindel and Blumberg, "Environmental Obesogens."
50. Environmental Working Group, "EWG's Tips to Avoid BPA Exposure," May 28, 2009, https://www.ewg.org/news-insights/news/ewgs-tips-avoid-bpa-exposure.
51. Luke Curtis, "Low- to Moderate-Level Chemical Exposures Can Trigger Migraines and Are Associated with Multiple Chemical Sensitivity," *Journal of Occupational Health* 64, no. 1 (July 2022): e12348, https://doi.org/10.1002%2F1348-9585.12348.
52. Vasundhara Aggarwal et al., "Environmental Toxins and Brain: Life on Earth Is in Danger," *Annals of Indian Academy of Neurology* 25, no. 1 (September 2022): S15–S21, https://doi.org/10.4103%2Faian.aian_169_22.
53. Ibid.
54. Bruno Bonaz, Thomas Bazin, and Sonia Pellissier, "The Vagus Nerve at the Interface of the Microbiota-Gut-Brain Axis," *Frontiers in Neuroscience* 12 (February 2018): 49, https://doi.org/10.3389%2Ffnins.2018.00049.
55. Karen Chiu et al., "The Impact of Environmental Chemicals on the Gut Microbiome," *Toxicological Sciences* 176, no. 2 (August 2020): 253–84, https://doi.org/10.1093%2Ftoxsci%2Fkfaa065.
56. Mondona S. McCann and Kathleen A. Maguire-Zeiss, "Environmental Toxicants in the Brain: A Review of Astrocytic Metabolic Dysfunction," *Environmental Toxicology and Pharmacology* 84 (May 2021): 103608, https://doi.org/10.1016/j.etap.2021.103608.

57. Aisha S. Dickerson et al., "A Scoping Review of Non-Occupational Exposures to Environmental Pollutants and Adult Depression, Anxiety, and Suicide," *Current Environmental Health Reports* 7, no. 3 (September 2020): 256–71, https://doi.org/10.1007/s40572-020-00280-7.
58. Parkinson's Foundation, "Environmental Factors," https://www.parkinson.org/understanding-parkinsons/causes/environmental-factors.
59. Yegambaram Manivannan et al., "Role of Environmental Contaminants in the Etiology of Alzheimer's Disease: A Review," *Current Alzheimer Research* 12, no. 2 (February 2015): 116–46, https://doi.org/10.2174%2F1567205012666150204121719.
60. Curtis, "Low-to Moderate-Level Chemical Exposures Can Trigger Migraines."
61. Megan Angelo, "16 Unforgettable Things Maya Angelou Wrote and Said," *Glamour*, May 28, 2014, https://www.glamour.com/story/maya-angelou-quotes.
62. Physicians for Social Responsibility, "Prenatal Exposure to Toxic Chemicals," https://www.psr.org/wp-content/uploads/2018/05/prenatal-exposure-to-chemicals.pdf.
63. Environmental Working Group, "Body Burden: The Pollution in Newborns," July 14, 2005, https://www.ewg.org/research/body-burden-pollution-newborns.
64. Natasha B. Scott and Nicola S. Pocock, "The Health Impacts of Hazardous Chemical Exposures among Child Labourers in Low- and Middle-Income Countries," *International Journal of Environmental Research and Public Health* 18, no. 10 (May 2021): 5496, https://doi.org/10.3390/ijerph18105496.
65. Cohen and vom Saal, *Non-Toxic*.
66. Environmental Working Group, "Understanding Skin Deep Ratings," https://www.ewg.org/skindeep/understanding_skin_deep_ratings/.
67. Environmental Protection Agency, "Contaminants in Schools and Child Care Facilities," https://www.epa.gov/americaschildrenenvironment/supplementary-topics-contaminants-schools-and-child-care-facilities.
68. Brenda D. Koester et al., "What Do Childcare Providers Know About Environmental Influences on Children's Health? Implications for Environmental Health Literacy Efforts," *International Journal of Environmental Research and Public Health* 18, no. 10 (May 2021): 5489, https://doi.org/10.3390%2Fijerph18105489.
69. Vera A. Paulson, Erin R. Rudzinski, and Douglas S. Hawkins, "Thyroid Cancer in the Pediatric Population," *Genes* (Basel) 10, no. 9 (September 2019): 723, https://www.ncbi.nlm.nih.gov/pmc/articles/PMC6771006/.
70. Elvira V. Brauner et al., "Trends in the Incidence of Central Precocious Puberty and Normal Variant Puberty among Children in Denmark, 1998 to 2017," *JAMA Network Open* 3, no. 10 (October 2020): e2015665, https://doi.org/10.1001/jamanetworkopen.2020.15665.
71. University of California Berkeley, "HERMOSA Study," https://cerch.berkeley.edu/research-programs/hermosa-study.
72. L. Levine and J. E. Hall, "Does the Environment Affect Menopause? A Review of the Effects of Endocrine Disrupting Chemicals on Menopause," *Climacteric* 26, no. 3 (June 2023): 206–15, https://doi.org/10.1080/13697137.2023.2173570.
73. Alison M. Neff et al., "The Effects of Environmental Contaminant Exposure on Reproductive Aging and the Menopause Transition," *Current Environmental Health Report* 9, no. 1 (February 2022): 53–79, https://doi.org/10.1007%2Fs40572-022-00334-y.
74. Paola Rebuzzini et al., "Multi- and Transgenerational Effects of Environmental Toxicants on Mammalian Reproduction," *Cells* 11, no. 19 (October 2022): 3163, https://doi.org/10.3390%2Fcells11193163.

75. Eric E. Nilsson, Millissia Ben Maamar, and Michael K Skinner, "Role of Epigenetic Transgenerational Inheritance in Generational Toxicology," *Environmental Epigenetics* 8, no.1 (February 2022), https://doi.org/10.1093/eep/dvac001.
76. Retha R. Newbold, "Lessons Learned from Perinatal Exposure to Diethylstilbestrol," *Toxicology and Applied Pharmacology* 199, no. 2 (September 2004): 142–50, https://doi.org/10.1016/j.taap.2003.11.033.
77. Umair Akbar et al., "Omega-3 Fatty Acids in Rheumatic Diseases: A Critical Review," *Journal of Clinical Rheumatology* 23, no. 6 (September 2017): 330–39, https://journals.lww.com/jclinrheum/fulltext/2017/09000/omega_3_fatty_acids_in_rheumatic_diseases__a.6.aspx.
78. Xinghua Gao et al., "Chronic Stress Promotes Colitis by Disturbing the Gut Microbiota and Triggering Immune System Response," *Proceedings of the National Academy of Sciences of the United States of America* 115, no. 13 (March 2018): E2960–E2969, https://doi.org/10.1073/pnas.1720696115.
79. Amber L. Simmons, Jennifer J. Schlezinger, and Barbara E. Corkey, "What Are We Putting in Our Food That Is Making Us Fat? Food Additives, Contaminants, and Other Putative Contributors to Obesity," *Current Obesity Reports* 3, no. 2 (June 2014): 273–85, https://doi.org/10.1007%2Fs13679-014-0094-y.

Chapter 3: How and Why Dangerous Environmental Chemicals Exist

1. David Andrews, "How American Industry Skips Some Chemical Safety Checks," Environmental Working Group, April 14, 2015, https://www.ewg.org/news-insights/news/how-american-industry-skips-some-chemical-safety-checks.
2. Melanie Benesh, "2 Years after Reformed TSCA, Pruitt's EPA Has Failed to Protect Us from Toxic Chemicals," Environmental Working Group, June 22, 2018, https://www.ewg.org/news-insights/news/2-years-after-reformed-tsca-pruitts-epa-has-failed-protect-us-toxic-chemicals.
3. US Government Accountability Office, "EPA Chemical Reviews," February 17, 2023, https://www.gao.gov/products/gao-23-105728.
4. Lillian Zhou and Julia Martiner, "Personal Care Product Chemicals Banned in Europe but Still Found in U.S.," Environmental Working Group, October 25, 2022, https://www.ewg.org/news-insights/news/2022/10/personal-care-product-chemicals-banned-europe-still-found-us.
5. European Environmental Bureau, "The Great Detox—Largest Ever Ban of Toxic Chemicals Announced by EU," April 25, 2022, https://eeb.org/the-great-detox-largest-ever-ban-of-toxic-chemicals-announced-by-eu/.
6. Steve Armstrong and George E. Dunaif, "Food Additive Reform: Time to Repeal the Delaney Clause?" Food & Drug Law Institute, https://www.fdli.org/2019/02/food-additive-reform-time-to-repeal-the-delaney-clause/.
7. Karen Selby, "20 Years Later: The Lingering Health Effects of 9/11," Asbestos.com, https://www.asbestos.com/featured-stories/9-11-lingering-health-effects.
8. Pew Charitable Trust, "Fixing the Oversight of Chemicals Added to Our Food," November 7, 2013, https://www.pewtrusts.org/en/research-and-analysis/reports/2013/11/07/fixing-the-oversight-of-chemicals-added-to-our-food.
9. Kristi Pullen Fedinick, "Millions Served by Water Systems Detecting Lead," Natural Resources Defense Council, May 13, 2021, https://www.nrdc.org/resources/millions-served-water-systems-detecting-lead.
10. Ravi Naidu et al., "Chemical Pollution: A Growing Peril and Potential

Catastrophic Risk to Humanity," *Environmental International* 156 (November 2021): 106616, https://doi.org/10.1016/j.envint.2021.106616.
11. Oluwademilade Fayemiwo and Kirsty Carden, "Emerging Contaminants: Approaches for Policy and Regulatory Responses in Low-Income Countries," in Willis Gwenzi, ed., *Emerging Contaminants in the Terrestrial-Aquatic-Atmosphere Continuum: Occurrence, Health Risks and Mitigation* (Amsterdam: Elsevier, 2022): 343–52, https://doi.org/10.1016/B978-0-323-90051-5.00010-9.
12. Environmental Working Group, "State of American Drinking Water," November 2021, https://www.ewg.org/tapwater/state-of-american-drinking-water.php.
13. Ibid.
14. Mark Scialla, "It Could Take Centuries for EPA to Test All the Unregulated Chemicals Under a New Landmark Bill," PBS News, June 22, 2016, https://www.pbs.org/newshour/science/it-could-take-centuries-for-epa-to-test-all-the-unregulated-chemicals-under-a-new-landmark-bill.
15. Jared Hayes, "For Decades, Polluters Knew PFAS Chemicals Were Dangerous but Hid Risks from Public," Environmental Working Group, August 29, 2019, https://www.ewg.org/research/decades-polluters-knew-pfas-chemicals-were-dangerous-hid-risks-public.
16. Ilaria Cimmino et al., "Potential Mechanisms of Bisphenol A (BPA) Contributing to Human Disease," *International Journal of Molecular Sciences* 21, no. 16 (August 2020): 5761, https://doi.org/10.3390%2Fijms21165761.
17. Michael Thoene et al., "Bisphenol S in Food Causes Hormonal and Obesogenic Effects Comparable to or Worse than Bisphenol A: A Literature Review," *Nutrients* 12, no. 2 (February 2020): 532, https://doi.org/10.3390%2Fnu12020532.
18. Stephen S. Hecht and Dorothy K. Hatsukami, "Smokeless Tobacco and Cigarette Smoking: Chemical Mechanisms and Cancer Prevention," *Nature Reviews Cancer* 22, no. 3 (2022): 143–55, https://doi.org/10.1038/s41568-021-00423-4.
19. F. R. de Gruijl, "Skin Cancer and Solar UV Radiation," *European Journal of Cancer* 35, no. 14 (1999): 2,003–9.
20. David Q. Andrews and Olga V. Naidenko, "Population-Wide Exposure to Per- and Polyfluoroalkyl Substances from Drinking Water in the United States," *Environmental Science & Technology Letters* 7, no. 12 (October 2020): 931–36, https://doi.org/10.1021/acs.estlett.0c00713.
21. Green Science Policy Institute, "Flame Retardants," https://greensciencepolicy.org/harmful-chemicals/flame-retardants/.
22. Thays Millena Alves Pedroso et al., "Cancer and Occupational Exposure to Pesticides: A Bibliometric Study of the Past 10 Years," *Environmental Science and Pollution Research* 29, no. 12 (October 2022): 17,464–75, https://doi.org/10.1007%2Fs11356-021-17031-2.
23. Peter L. deFur and Michelle Kaszuba, "Implementing the Precautionary Principle," *Science of the Total Environment* 288, nos. 1–2 (April 2002): 155–65, https://doi.org/10.1016/s0048-9697(01)01107-x.

Chapter 4: What's Really in Your Water

1. Kevin Varley, "NYC Is World's Wealthiest City, Bay Area Boasts Most Billionaires," *Bloomberg*, April 18, 2023, https://www.bloomberg.com/news/articles/2023-04-18/us-tops-china-australia-with-10-of-the-world-s-richest-cities.

2. "Arsenic Exposure Profile, Urine," Labcorp, https://www.labcorp.com/tests/007045/arsenic-exposure-profile-urine.
3. Kristi Pullen Fedinick, Mae Wu, and Erik D. Olson, "Threats on Tap: Widespread Violations Highlight Need for Investment in Water Infrastructure and Protections," Natural Resources Defense Council, May 2, 2017, https://www.nrdc.org/resources/threats-tap-widespread-violations-water-infrastructure.
4. Environmental Working Group, "Mapping the PFAS Contamination Crisis: New Data Show 7,457 Sites in 50 States, the District of Columbia and Four Territories," August 9, 2024, https://www.ewg.org/interactive-maps/pfas_contamination/.
5. Tatum Pied, "Bottled Water: The Human Health Consequences of Drinking from Plastic," Clean Water Action, July 29, 2020, https://cleanwater.org/2020/07/29/bottled-water-human-health-consequences-drinking-plastic.
6. Dana G. Smith, "How Much Can a Water Filter Do?" *New York Times*, May 30, 2023, https://www.nytimes.com/2023/05/30/well/live/water-filter-bacteria-pfas.html.
7. Ibid.
8. Ibid.
9. Li Lin, Haoran Yang, and Xiaocang Xu, "Effects of Water Pollution on Human Health and Disease Heterogeneity: A Review," *Frontiers in Environmental Science* 10 (June 2022), https://doi.org/10.3389/fenvs.2022.880246.
10. Environmental Protection Agency, "Indoor Water Use in the United States," June 2008, https://www.epa.gov/sites/default/files/2017-03/documents/ws-factsheet-indoor-water-use-in-the-us.pdf.
11. Barry M. Popkin, Kristen E. D'Anci, and Irwin H. Rosenberg, "Water, Hydration, and Health," *Nutrition Reviews* 68, no. 8 (August 2010): 439–58, https://doi.org/10.1111/j.1753-4887.2010.00304.x.
12. Ana-Maria Oros-Peusquens et al., "A Single-Scan, Rapid Whole-Brain Protocol for Quantitative Water Content Mapping with Neurobiological Implications," *Frontiers in Neurology* 10 (December 2019), https://doi.org/10.3389/fneur.2019.01333.
13. Melissa Denchak, "Water Pollution: Everything You Need to Know," Natural Resources Defense Council, January 11, 2023, https://www.nrdc.org/stories/water-pollution-everything-you-need-know.
14. Christopher P. Weis and Donald E. Tillitt, "Chemical Water Pollution and Human Health," in Aly Cohen et al., eds., *Integrative Environmental Medicine* (Oxford, UK: Oxford University Press, 2017), 87–114, https://doi.org/10.1093/med/9780190490911.003.0005.
15. Michael Birnbaum, "Desalination Can Make Saltwater Drinkable—But It Won't Solve the U.S. Water Crisis," *Washington Post*, September 28, 2021, https://www.washingtonpost.com/climate-solutions/2021/09/28/desalination-saltwater-drought-water-crisis/.
16. US Bureau of Reclamation, "Water Facts—Worldwide Water Supply," November 4, 2020, https://www.usbr.gov/mp/arwec/water-facts-ww-water-sup.html.
17. Denchak, "Water Pollution."
18. Environmental Protection Agency, "Nutrient Pollution: The Problem," https://www.epa.gov/nutrientpollution/problem.
19. "Toxicity of Industrial Water Pollution Underestimated," *Science Daily*, November 18, 2007, https://www.sciencedaily.com/releases/2007/11/071110081909.htm.

20. Utah State University, "How to Protect Your Water from Spilled Fuel," March 2012, https://digitalcommons.usu.edu/cgi/viewcontent.cgi?article=2201&context=extension_curall.
21. Andrew Hartsig and Chris Robbins, "*Exxon Valdez*: 29 Years Later," Ocean Conservancy, blog, March 22, 2018, https://oceanconservancy.org/blog/2018/03/22/exxon-valdez-29-years-later/.
22. Environmental Protection Agency, "Primer for Municipal Wastewater Treatment Systems," September 2004, https://www3.epa.gov/npdes/pubs/primer.pdf.
23. Environmental Protection Agency, "How Wastewater Treatment Works," May 1998, https://www3.epa.gov/npdes/pubs/bastre.pdf.
24. Aly Cohen and Frederick vom Saal, *Non-Toxic: Guide to Living Healthy in a Chemical World* (Oxford, UK: Oxford University Press, 2020).
25. Sydney Evans et al., "PFAS Contamination of Drinking Water Far More Prevalent Than Previously Reported," Environmental Working Group, January 23, 2020, https://www.ewg.org/research/national-pfas-testing.
26. Ian T. Cousins et al., "Outside the Safe Operating Space of a New Planetary Boundary for Per- and Polyfluoroalkyl Substances (PFAS)," *Environmental Science and Technology* 56, no. 16 (August 2022): 11,172–79, https://doi.org/10.1021/acs.est.2c02765.
27. Environmental Protection Agency, "Drinking Water Regulations," November 30, 2023, https://www.epa.gov/dwreginfo/drinking-water-regulations.
28. Environmental Working Group, "State of American Drinking Water," November 2021, https://www.ewg.org/tapwater/state-of-american-drinking-water.php.
29. Centers for Disease Control and Prevention, "Per- and Polyfluoroalkyl Substances (PFAS)," September 15, 2022, https://www.cdc.gov/niosh/topics/pfas/default.html; and California Department of Toxic Substances Control, "Chemicals of Emerging Concern," https://dtsc.ca.gov/emerging-chemicals-of-concern/.
30. Environmental Working Group, "PFAS Contamination in the U.S.," August 9, 2024, https://www.ewg.org/interactive-maps/pfas_contamination/.
31. Environmental Working Group, "State of American Drinking Water."
32. Ibid.
33. Daniel Eyal, "EPA's Lead and Copper Rule: Examining Challenges and Prospects," Environmental and Energy Law Program, January 28, 2021, https://eelp.law.harvard.edu/lead-and-copper-rule/.
34. Kristi Pullen Fedinick, "Millions Served by Water Systems Detecting Lead," Natural Resources Defense Council, May 13, 2021, https://www.nrdc.org/resources/millions-served-water-systems-detecting-lead.
35. Amanda MacMillan, "Safe Drinking Water," Natural Resources Defense Council, May 2, 2017, https://www.nrdc.org/stories/whats-your-drinking-water.
36. James McBride and Noah Berman, "How U.S. Water Infrastructure Works," Council on Foreign Relations, May 2, 2024, https://www.cfr.org/backgrounder/how-us-water-infrastructure-works.
37. National Cancer Institute, "Vinyl Chloride," June 13, 2024, https://www.cancer.gov/about-cancer/causes-prevention/risk/substances/vinyl-chloride.
38. "Report: The Perils of PVC Plastic Pipes," Beyond Plastics, April 2023, https://www.beyondplastics.org/publications/perils-of-pvc-pipes.
39. Environmental Working Group, "Plumbing & Pipes," https://www.ewg.org/healthyhomeguide/plumbing-and-pipes/.
40. Ibid.
41. National Centers of Environmental Information, "Tracking Global Marine Mi-

croplastics," August 17, 2022, https://www.ncei.noaa.gov/news/tracking-global-marine-microplastics.
42. Pennsylvania State University, "Microplastics in Our Waters, an Unquestionable Concern," Penn State Extension, August 26, 2022, https://extension.psu.edu/microplastics-in-our-waters-an-unquestionable-concern.
43. Suvash C. Saha and Goutam Saha, "Effect of Microplastics Deposition on Human Lung Airways: A Review with Computational Benefits and Challenges," *Heliyon* 10, no. 2 (January 2024): e24355, https://doi.org/10.1016%2Fj.heliyon.2024.e24355.
44. Margaret Osborne, "In a First, Microplastics Are Found in Fresh Antarctic Snow," *Smithsonian*, June 16, 2022, https://www.smithsonianmag.com/smart-news/in-a-first-microplastics-are-found-in-fresh-antarctic-snow-180980264/.
45. "Scientists Find Microplastics in Blood for First Time," Phys.org, March 25, 2022, https://phys.org/news/2022-03-scientists-microplastics-blood.html.
46. Raffaele Marfella et al., "Microplastics and Nanoplastics in Atheromas and Cardiovascular Events," *New England Journal of Medicine* 390, no. 10 (March 2024): 900–910, https://doi.org/10.1056/nejmoa2309822.
47. Louis Lloyd, "Microplastics in the Penis," *Nature Reviews Urology* 57 (July 2024), https://doi.org/10.1038/s41585-024-00917-4.
48. Qiancheng Zhao et al., "Detection and Characterization of Microplastics in the Human Testis and Semen," *Science of the Total Environment* 877 (June 2023): 162713, https://doi.org/10.1016/j.scitotenv.2023.162713.
49. Anne Pinto-Rodrigues, "Microplastics Are in Our Bodies. Here's Why We Don't Know the Health Risks," *Science News*, March 24, 2023, https://www.sciencenews.org/article/microplastics-human-bodies-health-risks.
50. Matthew Campen et al., "Bioaccumulation of Microplastics in Decedent Human Brains Assessed by Pyrolysis Gas Chromatography–Mass Spectrometry," *Research Square* preprint (May 2024), https://doi.org/10.21203/rs.3.rs-4345687/v1.
51. Pinto-Rodrigues, "Microplastics Are in Our Bodies."
52. Stephanie Schlea, "California Approves World's First Testing Requirement for Microplastics in Drinking Water," Association of State Drinking Water Administrators, September 9, 2022, https://www.asdwa.org/2022/09/09/california-approves-worlds-first-testing-requirement-for-microplastics-in-drinking-water/.
53. Water Resources Mission Area, "Domestic (Private) Supply Wells," US Geological Survey, March 1, 2019, https://www.usgs.gov/mission-areas/water-resources/science/domestic-private-supply-wells.
54. Ibid.
55. Centers for Disease Control and Prevention, "Guidelines for Testing Well Water," July 1, 2024, https://www.cdc.gov/drinking-water/safety/guidelines-for-testing-well-water.html.
56. Environmental Protection Agency, "Protect Your Home's Water," February 8, 2024, https://www.epa.gov/privatewells/protect-your-homes-water.
57. Centers for Disease Control and Prevention, "Community Water Fluoridation," https://www.cdc.gov/fluoridation/index.html.
58. Marge Dwyer, "A Call for Reducing Fluoride Levels in Drinking Water," March 10, 2015, https://www.hsph.harvard.edu/news/features/a-call-for-reducing-fluoride-levels-in-drinking-water/.
59. Centers for Disease Control and Prevention, "Community Water Fluoridation: Frequently Asked Questions," May 15, 2024, https://www.cdc.gov/fluoridation/faq/?CDC_AAref_Val=https://www.cdc.gov/fluoridation/faqs/wellwater.htm.
60. Zoreh Kheradpisheh et al., "Impact of Drinking Water Fluoride on Human

Thyroid Hormones: A Case-Control Study," *Scientific Reports* 8, no. 1 (February 2018): 2674, https://doi.org/10.1038%2Fs41598-018-20696-4.
61. Anna L. Choi et al., "Developmental Fluoride Neurotoxicity: A Systematic Review and Meta-Analysis," *Environmental Health Perspectives* 120, no. 10 (October 2012): 1,362–68, https://doi.org/10.1289%2Fehp.1104912.
62. A. Aravind et al., "Effect of Fluoridated Water on Intelligence in 10–12-Year-Old School Children," *Journal of International Society of Preventive and Community Dentistry* 6, no. 3 (December 2016): S237–S242, https://doi.org/10.4103%2F2231-0762.197204.
63. Tom C. Russ et al., "Aluminium and Fluoride in Drinking Water in Relation to Later Dementia Risk," *British Journal of Psychiatry* 216, no. 1 (January 2020): 29–34, doi: 10.1192/bjp.2018.287.
64. Nicole Davis, "Is Fluoridated Drinking Water Safe?" *Harvard Public Health*, https://www.hsph.harvard.edu/magazine/magazine_article/fluoridated-drinking-water/.
65. Amanda MacMillan, "Safe Drinking Water," Natural Resources Defense Council, May 2, 2017, https://www.nrdc.org/stories/whats-your-drinking-water.
66. Rae Lynn Mitchell, "Chlorine May Purify Drinking Water, but What Does It Leave Behind?" *Texas A&M Today*, March 31, 2017, https://vitalrecord.tamu.edu/chlorine-may-purify-drinking-water-but-what-does-it-leave-behind/.
67. Environmental Working Group, "Top 5 Reasons to Choose Filters over Bottled Water," November 2021, https://www.ewg.org/tapwater/bottled-water-resources.php; and Natural Resources Defense Council, "Bottled Water vs. Tap Water," September 13, 2023, https://www.nrdc.org/stories/truth-about-tap.
68. David Common and Eric Szeto, "Microplastics Found in 93% of Bottled Water Tested in Global Study," Canadian Broadcasting Corporation, March 14, 2018, https://www.cbc.ca/news/science/bottled-water-microplastics-1.4575045.
69. Environmental Working Group, "Top 5 Reasons to Choose Filters over Bottled Water."
70. Minnesota Department of Health, "Bottled Water: Questions and Answers," October 3, 2022, https://www.health.state.mn.us/communities/environment/water/factsheet/bottledwater.html.
71. Sytonia Reid, "Bottled Water vs. Tap: Which Is Best?" Green America, March 2024, https://www.greenamerica.org/drinking-water-risk/bottled-water-vs-tap-which-best.
72. Ibid.
73. Ryan Felton, "What's Really in Your Bottled Water?" *Consumer Reports*, September 24, 2020, https://www.consumerreports.org/water-quality/whats-really-in-your-bottled-water-a5361150329/.
74. Ibid.
75. Environmental Working Group, "Harmful Chemicals Found in Bottled Water," October 15, 2008, https://www.ewg.org/news-insights/news-release/harmful-chemicals-found-bottled-water.
76. Minnesota Department of Health, "Bottled Water."
77. Paul M. Bradley et al., "Bottled Water Contaminant Exposures and Potential Human Effects," *Environment International* 171 (January 2023): 107701, https://doi.org/10.1016/j.envint.2022.107701.
78. Environmental Working Group, "Top 5 Reasons to Choose Filters over Bottled Water."
79. "Bottled Water Is 3,500 Times Worse for the Environment than Tap Water, Say Scientists," *Euronews*, May 8, 2021, https://www.euronews.com/green/2021/08

/05/bottled-water-is-3-500-times-worse-for-the-environment-than-tap-water-say-scientists.
80. Rachel Ramirez, "The Plastic Water Bottle Industry Is Booming. Here's Why That's a Huge Problem," CNN, March 16, 2023, https://www.cnn.com/2023/03/16/world/plastic-water-bottles-un-report-climate/index.html.
81. American Cancer Society, "Arsenic and Cancer Risk," June 1, 2023, https://www.cancer.org/cancer/risk-prevention/chemicals/arsenic.html.
82. World Health Organization, "Arsenic," December 7, 2022, https://www.who.int/news-room/fact-sheets/detail/arsenic.
83. Ibid.
84. Joh Pujol, "What Do Brita Pitchers Filter Out?" Tap Score, *Tips for Taps* (blog), May 14, 2024, https://mytapscore.com/blogs/tips-for-taps/what-do-brita-pitchers-filter-out.
85. Ryan Felton, "Arsenic in Some Bottled Water Brands at Unsafe Levels, *Consumer Reports* Says," *Consumer Reports*, June 28, 2019, https://www.consumerreports.org/water-quality/arsenic-in-some-bottled-water-brands-at-unsafe-levels-a1198655241/.
86. Environmental Working Group, "Water Filter Technology: A Primer," August 2020, https://www.ewg.org/tapwater/water-filter-technology.php#ix.
87. Duke University, "Not All In-Home Drinking Water Filters Completely Remove Toxic PFAS," February 5, 2020, https://nicholas.duke.edu/news/not-all-home-drinking-water-filters-completely-remove-toxic-pfas.
88. "Do Water Softeners Remove Contaminants in Water?" C and J Water, September 16, 2022, https://candjwater.com/do-water-softeners-remove-contaminants-in-water/.
89. Environmental Working Group, "Water Filter Technology."
90. Duke University, "Not All In-Home Drinking Water Filters Completely Remove Toxic PFAS."
91. "Water Purity in Hemodialysis," Fresenius Medical Care, https://fmcna.com/insights/articles/importance-of-fluid-management-during-dialysis/.
92. US Customs and Border Protection, "Over 5,200 Fake Refrigerator Water Filters from China Seized by CBP at LA/Long Beach Seaport," September 30, 2019, https://www.cbp.gov/newsroom/local-media-release/over-5200-fake-refrigerator-water-filters-china-seized-cbp-lalong-beach.
93. National Sanitation Foundation, "Don't Be Fooled by Counterfeit Water Filters," May 24, 2022, https://www.nsf.org/news/dont-be-fooled-counterfeit-water-filters.
94. Water Quality Association, "Product Certification," https://wqa.org/grow/product-certification/.
95. Environmental Working Group, "Healthy Living Home Guide: Water Filters," https://www.ewg.org/healthyhomeguide/water-filters/.
96. Jorgen Stovne, "Is a Shower Filter Necessary?" Tap Score, January 5, 2020, https://mytapscore.com/blogs/tips-for-taps/is-a-shower-filter-necessary.
97. Dana G. Smith, "How Much Can a Water Filter Do?" *New York Times*, May 30, 2023, https://www.nytimes.com/2023/05/30/well/live/water-filter-bacteria-pfas.html.
98. City University of New York, "2019 Airline Water Study by CUNY's Hunter College NYC Food Policy Center," August 29, 2019, https://www.eurekalert.org/news-releases/602220.

Chapter 5: What's Really in Your Food

1. Kathleen L. Wyne et al., "Hypothyroidism Prevalence in the United States: A Retrospective Study Combining National Health and Nutrition Examination Survey and Claims Data, 2009–2019," *Journal of the Endocrine Society* 7, no. 1 (January 2023), https://doi.org/10.1210/jendso/bvac172.
2. National Institute of Diabetes and Digestive and Kidney Diseases, "Hashimoto's Disease," June 2021, https://www.niddk.nih.gov/health-information/endocrine-diseases/hashimotos-disease#common.
3. Karen Jesus Oliveira et al., "Thyroid Function Disruptors: From Nature to Chemicals," *Journal of Molecular Endocrinology* 62, no. 1 (January 2019): R1–R19, https://doi.org/10.1530/JME-18-0081.
4. Adrienne Hatch-McChesney and Harris R. Lieberman, "Iodine and Iodine Deficiency: A Comprehensive Review of a Re-Emerging Issue," *Nutrients* 14, no. 17 (August 2022): 3,474, https://doi.org/10.3390%2Fnu14173474.
5. J. L. Banach et al., "Cleaning and Disinfection in the Poultry, Eggs, Leafy Greens and Sprouts Supply Chains," Wageningen Food Safety Research, 2020, https://doi.org/10.18174/519367.
6. Maricel V. Maffini, Thomas G. Neltner, and Sarah Vogel, "We Are What We Eat: Regulatory Gaps in the United States that Put Our Health at Risk," *PLoS Biology* 15, no. 12 (December 2017): e2003578, https://doi.org/10.1371%2Fjournal.pbio.2003578.
7. Mary H. Ward et al., "Nitrate Intake and the Risk of Thyroid Cancer and Thyroid Disease," *Epidemiology* 21, no. 3 (May 2010): 389–95, https://doi.org/10.1097%2FEDE.0b013e3181d6201d.
8. Cecilie Bakken Høstmark, "A Mediterranean Diet Can Lead to a High Intake of Environmental Contaminants," University of Oslo, November 14, 2021, https://www.med.uio.no/imb/english/research/news-and-events/news/2021/mediterranean-diet-high-intake-of-contaminants.html.
9. Ibid.
10. Jessica Taylor Price, "Has Your Food Been Chemically Altered? New Database of 50,000 Products Provides Answers," *Northeastern Global News*, May 25, 2022, https://news.northeastern.edu/2022/05/25/ultra-processed-food-database/.
11. Maffini, Neltner, and Vogel, "We Are What We Eat."
12. Ibid.
13. Saseendran Sambu et al., "Toxicological and Teratogenic Effect of Various Food Additives: An Updated Review," *BioMed Research International* 2022, no. 1 (June 2022), https://doi.org/10.1155/2022/6829409.
14. Maffini, Neltner, and Vogel, "We Are What We Eat."
15. Ibid.
16. Pew Charitable Trust, "Fixing the Oversight of Chemicals Added to Our Food," November 7, 2013, https://www.pewtrusts.org/en/research-and-analysis/reports/2013/11/07/fixing-the-oversight-of-chemicals-added-to-our-food.
17. Ibid.
18. Olivia Backhaus and Melanie Benesh, "EWG Analysis: Almost All New Food Chemicals Greenlighted by Industry, not the FDA," Environmental Working Group, April 13, 2022, https://www.ewg.org/news-insights/news/2022/04/ewg-analysis-almost-all-new-food-chemicals-greenlighted-industry-not-fda.
19. Ibid.
20. Leonardo Trasande, Rachel M. Shaffer, and Sheela Sathyanarayana, "Food Ad-

ditives and Child Health," *Pediatrics* 142, no. 2 (December 2018): e20181408, https://doi.org/10.1542%2Fpeds.2018-1408.
21. Klara Matouskova, Thomas G. Neltner, and Maricel V. Maffini, "Out of Balance: Conflicts of Interest Persist in Food Chemicals Determined to Be Generally Recognized as Safe," *Environmental Health* 22, no. 1 (September 2023): 59, https://doi.org/10.1186/s12940-023-01004-8.
22. Alexis Temkin and Olga Naidenko, "Glyphosate Contamination in Food Goes Far Beyond Oat Products," Environmental Working Group, February 28, 2019, https://www.ewg.org/news-insights/news/2019/02/glyphosate-contamination-food-goes-far-beyond-oat-products.
23. Ibid.
24. "Genetically modified organisms—GMOs," MedlinePlus, July 30, 2022, https://medlineplus.gov/ency/article/002432.htm.
25. Aly Cohen and Frederick vom Saal, *Non-Toxic: Guide to Living Healthy in a Chemical World* (Oxford, UK: Oxford University Press, 2020).
26. Ibid.
27. Government of the Netherlands, "Antibiotic-Resistant Genes," https://www.government.nl/topics/biotechnology/antibiotic-resistant-genes.
28. A. S. Bawa and K. R. Anilakumar, "Genetically Modified Foods: Safety, Risks and Public Concerns—A Review," *Journal of Food Science and Technology* 50, no. 6 (December 2012): 1,035–46, https://doi.org/10.1007%2Fs13197-012-0899-1.
29. Laura Reiley, "The USDA's New Labeling for Genetically Modified Foods Goes into Effect Jan. 1. Here's What You Need to Know," *Washington Post*, January 1, 2022, https://www.washingtonpost.com/business/2022/01/01/usda-bioengineered-food-rules/.
30. "Seal: Non-GMO Project Verified," *Consumer Reports*, https://www.consumerreports.org/food-labels/seals-and-claims/non-gmo-project-verified.
31. US Department of Agriculture, "Recent Trends in GE Adoption," Economic Research Service, October 4, 2023, https://www.ers.usda.gov/data-products/adoption-of-genetically-engineered-crops-in-the-u-s/recent-trends-in-ge-adoption/.
32. Carol Potera, "Diet and Nutrition: The Artificial Food Dye Blues," *Environmental Health Perspectives* 118, no. 10 (October 2010): A428, https://doi.org/10.1289%2Fehp.118-a428.
33. Ibid.
34. Tasha Stoiber and Aurora Meadows, "California Agency Acknowledges Synthetic Food Dyes' Link to Hyperactivity and Behavioral Problems in Kids," Environmental Working Group, April 27, 2021, https://www.ewg.org/news-insights/news/2021/04/california-agency-acknowledges-synthetic-food-dyes-link-hyperactivity.
35. Dana G. Smith, "Two States Have Proposed Bans on Common Food Additives Linked to Health Concerns," *New York Times*, April 13, 2023, https://www.nytimes.com/2023/04/13/well/eat/food-additive-ban.html.
36. Aly Cohen and Frederick vom Saal, *Integrative Environmental Medicine* (Oxford, UK: Oxford University Press, 2017).
37. Iris Myers, "This Cancer-Causing Chemical May Be Lurking in Your Bread," Environmental Working Group, May 4, 2022, https://www.ewg.org/news-insights/news/2022/05/cancer-causing-chemical-may-be-lurking-your-bread.
38. Ketura Persellin and Melanie Benesh, "Watch for This Harmful Chemical in Your Soda," Environmental Working Group, January 13, 2021, https://www.ewg.org/news-insights/news/2021/01/watch-harmful-chemical-your-soda.

39. Smith, "Two States Have Proposed Bans on Common Food Additives."
40. Cohen and vom Saal, *Integrative Environmental Medicine.*
41. Ibid.
42. Smith, "Two States Have Proposed Bans on Common Food Additives."
43. Iris Myers, "EWG's Dirty Dozen Guide to Food Chemicals: The Top 12 to Avoid," Environmental Working Group, September 19, 2024, https://www.ewg.org/consumer-guides/ewgs-dirty-dozen-guide-food-chemicals-top-12-avoid.
44. "Whole food," *Cambridge Dictionary,* https://dictionary.cambridge.org/us/dictionary/english/whole-food.
45. Alisa Melse-Boonstra, "Bioavailability of Micronutrients from Nutrient-Dense Whole Foods: Zooming in on Dairy, Vegetables, and Fruits," *Frontiers in Nutrition* 7 (July 2020): 1,010, https://doi.org/10.3389%2Ffnut.2020.00101.
46. Center for Biological Diversity, "New Study: United States Uses 85 Pesticides Outlawed in Other Countries," June 6, 2019, https://biologicaldiversity.org/w/news/press-releases/united-states-uses-85-pesticides-outlawed-in-other-countries-2019-06-06/.
47. Yu-Han Chiu et al., "Comparison of Questionnaire-Based Estimation of Pesticide Residue Intake from Fruits and Vegetables with Urinary Concentrations of Pesticide Biomarkers," *Journal of Exposure Science and Environmental Epidemiology* 28, no. 1 (January 2018): 31–39, https://doi.org/10.1038%2Fjes.2017.22.
48. Gun-Hwi Lee and Kyung-Chul Choi, "Adverse Effects of Pesticides on the Functions of Immune System," *Comparative Biochemistry and Physiology, Part C: Toxicology & Pharmacology* 235 (September 2020): 108,789, https://doi.org/10.1016/j.cbpc.2020.108789.
49. Tianfang Jiang et al., "The Challenge of the Pathogenesis of Parkinson's Disease: Is Autoimmunity the Culprit?" *Frontiers in Immunology* 9 (September 2018): 20,147, https://doi.org/10.3389%2Ffimmu.2018.02047.
50. Vinay Mohan Pathak et al., "Current Status of Pesticide Effects on Environment, Human Health and Its Eco-Friendly Management as Bioremediation: A Comprehensive Review," *Frontiers in Microbiology* 13 (August 2022), https://doi.org/10.3389/fmicb.2022.962619.
51. Catherine Roberts, "Stop Eating Pesticides," *Consumer Reports,* August 27, 2020, https://www.consumerreports.org/health/food-contaminants/stop-eating-pesticides-a1094738355/.
52. Carly Hyland et al., "Organic Diet Intervention Significantly Reduces Urinary Pesticide Levels in U.S. Children and Adults," *Environmental Research* 171 (April 2019): 568–75, https://doi.org/10.1016/j.envres.2019.01.024.
53. Chiu et al., "Comparison of Questionnaire-Based Estimation of Pesticide Residue Intake."
54. Environmental Working Group, "These Four Foods Are High in Pesticides—Try Organic to Reduce Your Exposure," March 20, 2024, https://www.ewg.org/foodnews/five-lesser-known-foods-high-in-pesticides.php.
55. Carmen Costas-Ferreira, Rafael Duran, and Lilian R. F. Faro, "Toxic Effects of Glyphosate on the Nervous System: A Systematic Review," *International Journal of Molecular Sciences* 23, no. 9 (May 2022): 4,605, https://doi.org/10.3390%2Fijms23094605.
56. Walter J. Krol, "Removal of Trace Pesticide Residues from Produce," Connecticut Agricultural Experiment Station, https://portal.ct.gov/CAES/Fact-Sheets/Analytical-Chemistry/Removal-of-Trace-Pesticide-Residues-from-Produce.

57. Catherine Roberts, "An Easy Way to Remove Pesticides," *Consumer Reports*, October 25, 2017, https://www.consumerreports.org/pesticides-herbicides/easy-way-to-remove-pesticides-a3616455263/.
58. Mayo Clinic, "Organic Foods: Are They Safer? More Nutritious?" April 22, 2022, https://www.mayoclinic.org/healthy-lifestyle/nutrition-and-healthy-eating/in-depth/organic-food/art-20043880.
59. Cohen and vom Saal, *Non-Toxic*.
60. US Food and Drug Administration, "Chemical Contaminants," June 26, 2024, https://www.fda.gov/animal-veterinary/biological-chemical-and-physical-contaminants-animal-food/chemical-hazards.
61. Belachew B. Hirpessa, Beyza H. Ulusoy, and Canan Hecer, "Hormones and Hormonal Anabolics: Residues in Animal Source Food, Potential Public Health Impacts, and Methods of Analysis," *Journal of Food Quality* 2020, no. 1 (August 2020): 5065386, https://doi.org/10.1155/2020/5065386.
62. Gabriel K. Innes et al., "Contamination of Retail Meat Samples with Multidrug-Resistant Organisms in Relation to Organic and Conventional Production and Processing: A Cross-Sectional Analysis of Data from the United States National Antimicrobial Resistance Monitoring System, 2012–2017," *Environmental Health Perspectives* 129, no. 5 (May 2021), https://doi.org/10.1289/EHP7327.
63. Center for Food Safety, "Lawsuit Targets FDA Approval of Controversial Animal Drugs Used in Food Production," November 6, 2014, https://www.centerforfoodsafety.org/press-releases/3591/lawsuit-targets-fda-approval-of-controversial-animal-drugs-used-in-food-production.
64. Ibid.
65. US Department of Agriculture, "Never Fed Beta Agonists Program," Agricultural Marketing Service, https://www.ams.usda.gov/services/imports-exports/beta-agonists.
66. Washington State Department of Health, "Contaminants in Fish," https://doh.wa.gov/community-and-environment/food/fish/contaminants-fish.
67. Nadia Barbo et al., "Locally Caught Freshwater Fish across the United States Are Likely a Significant Source of Exposure to PFOS and Other Perfluorinated Compounds," *Environmental Research* 220 (March 2023): 115165, https://doi.org/10.1016/j.envres.2022.115165.
68. Luis Gabriel Antao Barboza et al., "Marine Microplastic Debris: An Emerging Issue for Food Security, Food Safety and Human Health," *Marine Pollution Bulletin* 133 (August 2018): 336–48, https://doi.org/10.1016/j.marpolbul.2018.05.047.
69. Plataforma SINC, "How to Remove Environmental Pollutants from Raw Meat," *Science Daily*, May 6, 2016, https://www.sciencedaily.com/releases/2016/05/160506100202.htm.
70. Julie Corliss, "Why Eat Lower on the Seafood Chain?" *Harvard Health Publishing*, March 22, 2023, https://www.health.harvard.edu/blog/why-eat-lower-on-the-seafood-chain-202303222904.
71. "Good News for Grilling: Black Pepper Helps Limit Cancerous Compounds in Meat, Study Shows," *K-State News*, May 16, 2017, https://www.k-state.edu/media/newsreleases/2017-05/grilling51617.html.
72. Cohen and vom Saal, *Non-Toxic*.
73. Lauren Kirchner and Althea Chang-Cook, "What Is Sustainable Seafood?" *Consumer Reports*, June 8, 2023, https://www.consumerreports.org/environment-sustainability/what-is-sustainable-seafood-a8919571798/.

74. Environmental Defense Fund, "Empowering Fishing Communities Worldwide," https://seafood.edf.org/guide/best.
75. Miles McEvoy, "Organic 101: What the USDA Organic Label Means," US Department of Agriculture blog, March 22, 2012, https://www.usda.gov/media/blog/2012/03/22/organic-101-what-usda-organic-label-means.
76. Mary Dunckel, Jeannine Schweihofer, and Ashley Kuschel, "Natural and Organic Label Claims," Michigan State University, September 30, 2020, https://www.canr.msu.edu/resources/natural-and-organic-label-claims.
77. "Seal: Non-GMO Project Verified."
78. US Department of Agriculture, "What Is 'Grass Fed' Meat?" April 16, 2024, https://ask.usda.gov/s/article/What-is-grass-fed-meat.
79. US Department of Agriculture, "Food Safety and Inspection Service Labeling Guideline on Documentation Needed to Substantiate Animal Raising Claims for Label Submissions," December 2019, https://www.fsis.usda.gov/sites/default/files/media_file/2021-02/RaisingClaims.pdf.
80. Trisha Calvo, "Cage-Free vs. Free Range—and Other Egg Carton Labels—Explained," *Consumer Reports*, January 31, 2023, https://www.consumerreports.org/health/food-labeling/egg-carton-labels-explained-a1022347027/.
81. US Department of Agriculture, "Does the Label 'Free Range' Pertain Only to Poultry or Also to Meats?" April 16, 2024, https://ask.usda.gov/s/article/Does-the-label-free-range-pertain-only-to-poultry-or-also-to-meats.
82. Ibid.
83. Birgit Geueke et al., "Systematic Evidence on Migrating and Extractable Food Contact Chemicals: Most Chemicals Detected in Food Contact Materials Are Not Listed for Use," *Critical Reviews in Food Science and Nutrition* 63, no. 28 (May 2022): 9,425–35, https://doi.org/10.1080/10408398.2022.2067828.
84. Ibid.
85. "Food Packaging Chemicals May Be Harmful to Human Health over Long Term," *Science Daily*, February 19, 2014, https://www.sciencedaily.com/releases/2014/02/140219205215.htm#google_vignette.
86. Jane Muncke et al., "Impacts of Food Contact Chemicals on Human Health: A Consensus Statement," *Environmental Health* 19, no. 25 (March 2020), https://doi.org/10.1186/s12940-020-0572-5.
87. Kevin Loria, "Dangerous PFAS Chemicals Are in Your Food Packaging," *Consumer Reports*, March 24, 2022, https://www.consumerreports.org/health/food-contaminants/dangerous-pfas-chemicals-are-in-your-food-packaging-a3786252074/.
88. US Food and Drug Administration, "FDA, Industry Actions End Sales of PFAS Used in U.S. Food Packaging," February 28, 2024, https://www.fda.gov/news-events/press-announcements/fda-industry-actions-end-sales-pfas-used-us-food-packaging.
89. Cohen and vom Saal, *Non-Toxic*.
90. Min Kyong Moon, "Concern About the Safety of Bisphenol A Substitutes," *Diabetes & Metabolism Journal* 43, no. 1 (February 2019): 46–48, https://doi.org/10.4093%2Fdmj.2019.0027.
91. Cohen and vom Saal, *Non-Toxic*.
92. Deborah Balthazar, Daniel Leonard, and Tatum McConnell, "Is it Safe to Microwave Plastic Containers?" *ScienceLine*, September 8, 2022, https://scienceline.org/2022/09/is-it-safe-to-microwave-plastic-containers/.
93. Cohen and vom Saal, *Non-Toxic*.
94. Laura M. Hernandez et al., "Plastic Teabags Release Billions of Microparticles

and Nanoparticles into Tea," *Environmental Science & Technology* 53, no. 21 (September 2019): 12,300–310, https://doi.org/10.1021/acs.est.9b02540.
95. Cohen and vom Saal, *Non-Toxic*.
96. Kevin Loria, "You Can't Always Trust Claims on 'Non-Toxic' Cookware," *Consumer Reports*, October 26, 2022, https://www.consumerreports.org/toxic-chemicals-substances/you-cant-always-trust-claims-on-non-toxic-cookware-a4849321487/.
97. Hillary L. Shane et al., "Topical Exposure to Triclosan Inhibits Th1 Immune Responses and Reduces T Cells Responding to Influenza Infection in Mice," *PLoS One* 15, no. 12 (December 2020): e0244436, https://doi.org/10.1371%2Fjournal.pone.0244436.
98. Katherine Quinn Newman and Charles Guy Castles, "Use of Doxycycline in a Patient Following Minocycline-Induced Lupus," *Case Reports in Rheumatology* 2023, no. 1 (July 2023): 7353644, https://doi.org/10.1155%2F2023%2F7353644.
99. Ye He and Amr H. Sawalha, "Drug-Induced Lupus Erythematosus: An Update on Drugs and Mechanisms," *Current Opinion in Rheumatology* 30, no. 5 (September 2018): 490–97, https://doi.org/10.1097%2FBOR.0000000000000522.
100. Lisa Maier et al., "Extensive Impact of Non-Antibiotic Drugs on Human Gut Bacteria," *Nature* 555, no. 7698 (2018): 623–28, https://doi.org/10.1038/nature25979.
101. Leyuan Li et al., "RapidAIM: A Culture- and Metaproteomics-Based Rapid Assay of Individual Microbiome Responses to Drugs," *Microbiome* 8, no. 33 (2020), https://doi.org/10.1186/s40168-020-00806-z.
102. Simona Bancos et al., "Ibuprofen and Other Widely Used Non-Steroidal Anti-Inflammatory Drugs Inhibit Antibody Production in Human Cells," *Cellular Immunology* 258, no. 1 (April 2009): 18–28, https://doi.org/10.1016%2Fj.cellimm.2009.03.007.
103. Cohen and vom Saal, *Non-Toxic*.
104. Zane R. Gallinger and Geoffrey C. Nguyen, "Presence of Phthalates in Gastrointestinal Medications: Is There a Hidden Danger?" *World Journal of Gastroenterology* 19, no. 41 (November 2013): 7,042–47, https://doi.org/10.3748%2Fwjg.v19.i41.7042.

Chapter 6: What's Really in Your Personal-Care Products

1. Jada Poole, "What Are Some of the Health Complications of Foot Binding?" MyMed.com, https://www.mymed.com/health-wellness/body-modifications/foot-binding/what-are-some-of-the-health-complications-of-foot-binding.
2. T. R. Forbes, "Why Is It Called 'Beautiful Lady'? A Note on Belladonna," *Bulletin of the New York Academy of Medicine* 53, no. 4 (May 1977): 403–6, https://www.ncbi.nlm.nih.gov/pmc/articles/PMC1807294/.
3. Fiona McNeill, "Analysis: Dying for Makeup—Lead Cosmetics Poisoned 18th-Century European Socialites in Search of Whiter Skin," McMaster University, February 28, 2022, https://brighterworld.mcmaster.ca/articles/analysis-dying-for-makeup-lead-cosmetics-poisoned-18th-century-european-socialites-in-search-of-whiter-skin/.
4. Jacopo Prisco, "When Beauty Products Were Radioactive," CNN, March 8, 2020, https://www.cnn.com/style/article/when-beauty-products-were-radioactive/index.html.

5. Aly Cohen and Frederick vom Saal, *Non-Toxic: Guide to Living Healthy in a Chemical World* (Oxford, UK: Oxford University Press, 2020).
6. Lisa Girion, "Johnson & Johnson Knew for Decades That Asbestos Lurked in Its Baby Powder," Reuters, December 14, 2018, https://www.reuters.com/investigates/special-report/johnsonandjohnson-cancer/.
7. Cohen and vom Saal, *Non-Toxic*.
8. Collaborative for Health & Environment, "Precautionary Principle: The Wingspread Statement," https://www.healthandenvironment.org/environmental-health/social-context/history/precautionary-principle-the-wingspread-statement.
9. Occupational Safety and Health Administration, "Health Hazards in Nail Salons," https://www.osha.gov/nail-salons.
10. Campaign for Safe Cosmetics, "Nail Polish Removers," https://www.safecosmetics.org/chemicals/nail-polish-removers/.
11. Scott Faber, "The Toxic Twelve Chemicals and Contaminants in Cosmetics," Environmental Working Group, https://www.ewg.org/the-toxic-twelve-chemicals-and-contaminants-in-cosmetics.
12. Environmental Working Group, "Hormone-Altering Cosmetics Chemicals Found in Teenage Girls," https://www.ewg.org/news-insights/news-release/hormone-altering-cosmetics-chemicals-found-teenage-girls.
13. Knvul Sheikh, "Many Personal Care Products Contain Harmful Chemicals. Here's What to Do About It," *New York Times*, February 15, 2023, https://www.nytimes.com/2023/02/15/well/live/personal-care-products-chemicals.html.
14. Faber, "The Toxic Twelve Chemicals and Contaminants in Cosmetics."
15. Ibid.
16. Laura N. Vandenberg et al., "Hormones and Endocrine-Disrupting Chemicals: Low-Dose Effects and Nonmonotonic Dose Responses," *Endocrine Reviews* 33, no. 3 (June 2012): 378–455, https://doi.org/10.1210/er.2011-1050.
17. Faber, "The Toxic Twelve Chemicals and Contaminants in Cosmetics."
18. Kimberly P. Berger et al., "Personal Care Product Use as a Predictor of Urinary Concentrations of Certain Phthalates, Parabens, and Phenols in the HERMOSA Study," *Journal of Exposure Science & Environmental Epidemiology* 29, no. 1 (January 2018): 21–32, https://doi.org/10.1038%2Fs41370-017-0003-z.
19. Faber, "The Toxic Twelve Chemicals and Contaminants in Cosmetics."
20. Ibid.
21. Ibid.
22. Environmental Working Group, "EWG Welcomes Cosmetics Law Reforms in End-of-Year Spending Bill," December 23, 2022, https://www.ewg.org/news-insights/news-release/2022/12/ewg-welcomes-cosmetics-law-reforms-end-year-spending-bill.
23. Cleveland Clinic, "Skin," https://my.clevelandclinic.org/health/articles/10978-skin.
24. Douglas Wilkin and Jean Brainard, *13.11 Skin*, FlexBooks, August 21, 2024, https://flexbooks.ck12.org/cbook/ck-12-biology-flexbook-2.0/section/13.11/primary/lesson/skin-bio/.
25. H. S. Brown, D. R. Bishop, and C. A. Rowan, "The Role of Skin Absorption as a Route of Exposure for Volatile Organic Compounds (VOCs) in Drinking Water," *American Journal of Public Health* 74, no. 5 (May 1984): 479–84, https://doi.org/10.2105%2Fajph.74.5.479.
26. Cohen and vom Saal, *Non-Toxic*.

27. Nina Otberg et al., "The Role of Hair Follicles in the Percutaneous Absorption of Caffeine," *British Journal of Clinical Pharmacology* 65, no. 4 (December 2007): 488–92, https://doi.org/10.1111%2Fj.1365-2125.2007.03065.x.
28. Faber, "The Toxic Twelve Chemicals and Contaminants in Cosmetics."
29. Sheikh, "Many Personal Care Products Contain Harmful Chemicals."
30. Nneka Leiba and Paul Pestano, "Study: Women of Color Exposed to More Toxic Chemicals in Personal Care Products," Environmental Working Group, August 17, 2017, https://www.ewg.org/news-insights/news/study-women-color-exposed-more-toxic-chemicals-personal-care-products.
31. Ami R. Zota and Bhavna Shamasunder, "The Environmental Injustice of Beauty: Framing Chemical Exposures from Beauty Products as a Health Disparities Concern," *American Journal of Obstetrics & Gynecology* 217, no. 4 (October 2017): 418.E1–418.E6, https://doi.org/10.1016/j.ajog.2017.07.020.
32. Campaign for Safe Cosmetics, "Non-Toxic Black Beauty Project," https://www.safecosmetics.org/black-beauty-project/.
33. Paula I. Johnson et al., "Chemicals of Concern in Personal Care Products Used by Women of Color in Three Communities of California," *Journal of Exposure Science & Environmental Epidemiology* 32 (November 2022): 864–76, https://doi.org/10.1038/s41370-022-00485-y.
34. Campaign for Safe Cosmetics, "Non-Toxic Black Beauty Project."
35. Breast Cancer Research Foundation, "Black Women and Breast Cancer: Why Disparities Persist and How to End Them," BCRF blog, February 7, 2024, https://www.bcrf.org/blog/black-women-and-breast-cancer-why-disparities-persist-and-how-end-them/.
36. "Formaldehyde and Cancer Risk," American Cancer Society, October 24, 2022, https://www.cancer.org/cancer/risk-prevention/chemicals/formaldehyde.html.
37. Cleveland Clinic, "Are Natural Skin Care Products Actually Better for Your Skin?" April 14, 2023, https://health.clevelandclinic.org/natural-skin-care/.
38. Cohen and vom Saal, *Non-Toxic*.
39. Sheikh, "Many Personal Care Products Contain Harmful Chemicals."
40. Cohen and vom Saal, *Non-Toxic*.
41. Environmental Working Group, "The Trouble with Ingredients in Sunscreens," https://www.ewg.org/sunscreen/report/the-trouble-with-sunscreen-chemicals/.
42. Center for Science in the Public Interest, "Watchdog Group to Consumers: Avoid Titanium Dioxide," December 5, 2022, https://www.cspinet.org/press-release/watchdog-group-consumers-avoid-titanium-dioxide.
43. Skin Cancer Foundation, "Skin Cancer Facts & Statistics," February 2024, https://www.skincancer.org/skin-cancer-information/skin-cancer-facts/.
44. Cohen and vom Saal, *Non-Toxic*.
45. Wendee Nicole, "A Question for Women's Health: Chemicals in Feminine Hygiene Products and Personal Lubricants," *Environmental Health Perspectives* 122, no. 3 (March 2014): A70–A75, https://doi.org/10.1289/ehp.122-A70.
46. Women's Voices for the Earth, "New Tampon Testing Reveals Undisclosed Carcinogens and Reproductive Toxins," June 5, 2018, https://womensvoices.org/2018/06/05/new-tampon-testing-reveals-undisclosed-carcinogens-and-reproductive-toxins/.
47. Jenni Shearston et al., "Tampons as a Source of Exposure to Metal(loid)s," *Environment International* 190 (2024): 108849, https://doi.org/10.1016/j.envint.2024.108849.

48. Caroline Linhart et al., "Use of Underarm Cosmetic Products in Relation to Risk of Breast Cancer: A Case-Control Study," *EBioMedicine* 21 (July 2017): 79–85, https://doi.org/10.1016/j.ebiom.2017.06.005.
49. P. D. Darbre, "Aluminium and the Human Breast," *Morphologie* 100, no. 329 (June 2016): 65–74, https://doi.org/10.1016/j.morpho.2016.02.001.
50. American Cancer Society, "Antiperspirants and Breast Cancer Risk," October 19, 2022, https://www.cancer.org/cancer/risk-prevention/chemicals/antiperspirants-and-breast-cancer-risk.html.

Chapter 7: What's Really Inside Your Home

1. For information on the world's Blue Zones, visit https://www.bluezones.com/.
2. Environmental Protection Agency, "Indoor Air Quality," July 14, 2023, https://www.epa.gov/report-environment/indoor-air-quality.
3. Aly Cohen and Frederick vom Saal, *Non-Toxic: Guide to Living Healthy in a Chemical World* (Oxford, UK: Oxford University Press, 2020).
4. Dana G. Smith, "You Don't Need to Disinfect So Much," *New York Times*, March 21, 2023, https://www.nytimes.com/2023/03/21/well/live/cleaning-disinfectant-bleach-risks.html.
5. Ibid.
6. Mon H. Tun et al., "Postnatal Exposure to Household Disinfectants, Infant Gut Microbiota and Subsequent Risk of Overweight in Children," *Canadian Medical Association Journal* 190, no. 37 (September 2018): E1097–E1107, https://doi.org/10.1503%2Fcmaj.170809.
7. Kim E. Andreassen, "Household Cleaning Can Be as Bad as Smoking for Lung Function," University of Bergen, February 16, 2018, https://www.uib.no/en/news/115228/household-cleaning-can-be-bad-smoking-lung-function.
8. Environmental Working Group Guide to Healthy Cleaning, "Secret Ingredients, Hidden Hazards," https://www.ewg.org/cleaners/content/secret-ingredients/.
9. Rebecca Trager, "US Agencies Test Less than 1% of Chemicals," Royal Society of Chemistry, November 30, 2015, https://www.chemistryworld.com/news/us-agencies-test-less-than-1-of-chemicals-/9220.article.
10. Per A. Clausen et al., "Chemicals Inhaled from Spray Cleaning and Disinfection Products and Their Respiratory Effects: A Comprehensive Review," *International Journal of Hygiene and Environmental Health* 229 (August 2020): 113592, https://www.sciencedirect.com/science/article/pii/S1438463920305381.
11. Environmental Working Group, "Understanding Skin Deep Ratings," https://www.ewg.org/skindeep/understanding_skin_deep_ratings/; and Marine Peyneau et al., "Quaternary Ammonium Compounds in Hypersensitivity Reactions," *Frontiers in Toxicology* 16, no. 4 (September 2022): 973680, https://doi.org/10.3389/ftox.2022.973680.
12. Allison Guy, "What Are Endocrine-Disrupting Chemicals?" Environmental Health News, July 26, 2023, https://www.ehn.org/what-are-endocrine-disrupting-chemicals-2662337230.html.
13. Environmental Working Group, Guide to Healthy Living, "Household Cleaner Ratings and Ingredients," https://www.ewg.org/cleaners/content/findings/.
14. Elaine K. Howley, "Do I Need to Worry About Household Cleaners and Cancer Risk?" *U.S. News & World Report*, July 18, 2018, https://health.usnews.com/health-care/patient-advice/articles/2018-07-18/do-i-need-to-worry-about-household-chemicals-and-cancer-risk.

15. Shao Lin et al., "Maternal Occupation and the Risk of Major Birth Defects: A Follow-Up Analysis from the National Birth Defects Prevention Study," *International Journal of Hygiene and Environmental Health* 216, no. 3 (November 2013), https://doi.org/10.1016%2Fj.ijheh.2012.05.006.
16. Kate Arcell, "News: Your Disinfectant Wipes Could Be Making You Fat, Foggy, and Tired—MDs Weigh In on the Health Dangers of 'Quats,'" First for Women, September 4, 2023, https://www.firstforwomen.com/posts/health/quaternary-ammonium-compounds.
17. Kelsey Oliver, "Potentially Carcinogenic Chemicals More Associated with Conventional Cleaning Products, but Also with Some 'Green' Products," Berkeley Public Health, January 3, 2023, https://publichealth.berkeley.edu/news-media/research-highlights/carcinogenic-chemicals-associated-with-both-traditional-and-green-cleaning-products/.
18. Environmental Working Group, "Green Works Laundry Detergent, Original," March 14, 2016, https://www.ewg.org/guides/cleaners/5169-GreenWorksLaundryDetergentOriginal/.
19. Environmental Working Group, "Scoring Substances & Products," https://www.ewg.org/cleaners/content/scoring/.
20. Environmental Working Group, "365 Everyday Value 2X Concentrated Liquid Laundry Detergent, Unscented," March 14, 2016, https://www.ewg.org/guides/cleaners/6408-365EverydayValue2XConcentratedLiquidLaundryDetergentUnscented/.
21. Cohen and vom Saal, *Non-Toxic*.
22. Environmental Working Group, "Guide to Healthy Cleaning," https://www.ewg.org/guides/cleaners/content/faq/#q6.
23. Lauren Smith McDonough and Alyssa Gautieri, "How to Make Simple Homemade Cleaning Sprays," *Good Housekeeping*, June 28, 2024, https://www.goodhousekeeping.com/home/cleaning/tips/a24885/make-at-home-cleaners/.
24. Cohen and vom Saal, *Non-Toxic*.
25. Environmental Working Group Guide to Healthy Cleaning, "Frequently Asked Questions," https://www.ewg.org/cleaners/content/faq/#q19.
26. Environmental Protection Agency, "Pesticides' Impact on Indoor Air Quality," https://www.epa.gov/indoor-air-quality-iaq/pesticides-impact-indoor-air-quality.
27. Environmental Working Group Guide to Healthy Cleaning, "Frequently Asked Questions."
28. Cohen and vom Saal, *Non-Toxic*.
29. Johanna Congleton, "Flame Retardants: Why They're in Our Homes and How to Avoid Them," Environmental Working Group, August 16, 2016, https://www.ewg.org/news-insights/news/flame-retardants-why-theyre-our-homes-and-how-avoid-them.
30. Rob Spahr, "New Study Reveals Unregulated Toxic Chemicals in Breast Milk," Emory University, August 9, 2023, https://news.emory.edu/stories/2023/08/hs_toxic_chemicals_breast_milk_09-08-2023/story.html.
31. Kim G. Harley et al., "PBDE Concentrations in Women's Serum and Fecundability," *Environmental Health Perspectives* 118, no. 5 (2010): 699–704, https://doi.org/10.1289/ehp.0901450.
32. Cohen and vom Saal, *Non-Toxic*.
33. Tom Perkins, "Toxic PFAS Not Necessary to Make Fabric Stain Repellent, Study Finds," *Guardian*, April 7, 2023, https://www.theguardian.com/environment/2023/apr/07/toxic-pfas-fabric-stain-water-repellent-study.

34. Ibid.
35. Hannah Norman, "Raincoats, Undies, School Uniforms: Are Your Clothes Dripping in 'Forever Chemicals'?" CBS News, March 30, 2023, https://www.cbsnews.com/news/pfas-in-clothing-household-items-consumer-products-forever-chemicals/.
36. Beyond Plastics, "Vinyl Chloride: A Toxic Chemical That Threatens Human Health," https://www.beyondplastics.org/fact-sheets/vinyl-chloride.
37. Matthew Daly, "EPA Weighs Formal Review of Vinyl Chloride, the Toxic Chemical That Burned in Ohio Train Derailment," AP News, August 11, 2023, https://apnews.com/article/vinyl-chloride-ohio-train-derailment-toxic-chemicals-54bb0a943f4f4af0e4f68cc60ce4edb4.
38. Minnesota Department of Health, "Formaldehyde in Your Home," October 3, 2022, https://www.health.state.mn.us/communities/environment/air/toxins/formaldehyde.htm.
39. Environmental Working Group, "Mattresses," https://www.ewg.org/healthyhomeguide/mattresses/.
40. Cohen and vom Saal, *Non-Toxic*.
41. James Miller, "How Long Does It Take for Furniture to Off-Gas?" Roundup, March 19, 2024, https://theroundup.org/how-long-does-it-take-for-furniture-to-off-gas/.
42. Cohen and vom Saal, *Non-Toxic*.
43. Ibid.
44. Environmental Working Group, "Carpet," https://www.ewg.org/healthyhomeguide/carpet/.
45. Earth Day, "Toxic Textiles: The Chemicals in Our Clothing," November 4, 2022, https://www.earthday.org/toxic-textiles-the-chemicals-in-our-clothing/.
46. Emily Difrisco, "New Testing Shows High Levels of BPA in Sports Bras and Athletic Shirts," Center for Environmental Health, October 12, 2022, https://ceh.org/latest/press-releases/new-testing-shows-high-levels-of-bpa-in-sports-bras-and-athletic-shirts/.
47. Earth Day, "Toxic Textiles."
48. Environmental Protection Agency, "Tetrachloroethylene (Perchloroethylene)," January 2000, https://www.epa.gov/sites/default/files/2016-09/documents/tetrachloroethylene.pdf.
49. Cohen and vom Saal, *Non-Toxic*.
50. Jing Ma et al., "Association between Residential Proximity to PERC Dry Cleaning Establishments and Kidney Cancer in New York City," *Journal of Environmental and Public Health* 2009, no. 1 (January 2010), https://doi.org/10.1155/2009/183920.
51. New York City Health Department, "Do You Live by a Dry Cleaner?" https://www.nyc.gov/assets/doh/downloads/pdf/environmental/air-tests-for-dry-cleaning-chemicals.pdf.
52. Cohen and vom Saal, *Non-Toxic*.

Chapter 8: Using Food to Detoxify

1. Oregon State University, "Micronutrient Inadequacies in the US Population: An Overview," https://lpi.oregonstate.edu/mic/micronutrient-inadequacies/overview.
2. Ghania Qureshi et al., "The Non-Conventional Effects of Hypovitaminosis D:

A Pandemic Even in Sunlight-Rich Countries," *Cureus* 16, no. 4 (April 2024): e59267, doi: 10.7759/cureus.59267.
3. Luoping Zhang et al., "Exposure to Glyphosate-Based Herbicides and Risk for Non-Hodgkin Lymphoma: A Meta-Analysis and Supporting Evidence," *Mutation Research/Reviews in Mutation Research* 781 (July–September 2019): 186–206, https://doi.org/10.1016/j.mrrev.2019.02.001/.
4. Clinical Applications of Scientific Intervention, "Cruciferous Vegetables to Promote Liver Detox," January 30, 2023, https://www.casi.org/cruciferous-vegetables-to-promote-liver-detox.
5. Breast Cancer Now, "Novel Drug Inspired by Cruciferous Vegetables Could Reverse Drug Resistance in Estrogen Receptor Positive Breast Cancer," January 27, 2020, https://breastcancernow.org/about-us/research-news/novel-drug-inspired-cruciferous-vegetables-could-reverse-drug-resistance-in-oestrogen-receptor-positive-breast-cancer/.
6. Marijke Jozefczak et al., "Glutathione Is a Key Player in Metal-Induced Oxidative Stress Defenses," *Internal Journal of Molecular Sciences* 13, no. 3 (March 2012): 3,145–75, https://doi.org/10.3390%2Fijms13033145.
7. Mark Hyman, "Glutathione: The Mother of All Antioxidants," *HuffPost*, June 10, 2010, https://www.huffpost.com/entry/glutathione-the-mother-of_b_530494.
8. Deanna M. Minich and Benjamin I. Brown, "A Review of Dietary (Phyto) Nutrients for Glutathione Support," *Nutrients* 11, no. 9 (September 2019): 2073, https://doi.org/10.3390%2Fnu11092073.
9. Chu Won Nho and Elizabeth Jeffery, "The Synergistic Upregulation of Phase II Detoxification Enzymes by Glucosinolate Breakdown Products in Cruciferous Vegetables," *Toxicology and Applied Pharmacology* 174, no. 2 (July 2001): 146–52, https://doi.org/10.1006/taap.2001.9207.
10. J. W. Fahey and P. Talalay, "Antioxidant Functions of Sulforaphane: A Potent Inducer of Phase II Detoxication Enzymes," *Food and Chemical Toxicology* 37, nos. 9–10 (October 1999): 973–79, https://doi.org/10.1016/S0278-6915(99)00082-4.
11. N. Kaplowitz, "The Importance and Regulation of Hepatic Glutathione," *Yale Journal of Biology and Medicine* 54, no. 6 (November–December 1981): 497–502, https://www.ncbi.nlm.nih.gov/pmc/articles/PMC2596047/.
12. John A. Bouranis et al., "Interplay between Cruciferous Vegetables and the Gut Microbiome: A Multi-Omic Approach," *Nutrients* 15, no. 1 (December 2022): 42, https://doi.org/10.3390%2Fnu15010042.
13. Melissa Matthews, "For Best Nutrition, Chop Broccoli into Small Pieces Before Cooking, Study Finds," *Newsweek*, February 9, 2018, https://www.newsweek.com/best-nutrition-chop-broccoli-small-pieces-cooking-study-finds-801712.
14. Mark Percival, "Phytonutrients & Detoxification," *Clinical Nutrition Insights* 5, no. 2 (1997): 1–4, https://www.acudoc.com/phytonutrients%20and%20detoxification.pdf.
15. Yahya Asemani et al., "Allium Vegetables for Possible Future of Cancer Treatment," *Phytotherapy Research* 33, no. 12 (December 2019): 3,019–39, https://doi.org/10.1002/ptr.6490.
16. Cleia Rocha de Oliveira et al., "Effects of Quercetin on Polychlorinated Biphenyls-Induced Liver Injury in Rats," *Nutricion Hospitalaria* 29, no. 5 (May 2014): 1,141–48, https://doi.org/10.3305/nh.2014.29.5.7362.
17. Damini Kothari, Woo-Do Lee, and Soo-Ki Kim, "*Allium* Flavonols: Health Benefits, Molecular Targets, and Bioavailability," *Antioxidants* 9, no. 9 (September 2020): 888, https://doi.org/10.3390%2Fantiox9090888.

18. Yupei Deng et al., "Bioavailability, Health Benefits, and Delivery Systems of Allicin: A Review," *Journal of Agricultural and Food Chemistry* 71, no. 49 (December 2023): 19,207–20, https://doi.org/10.1021/acs.jafc.3c05602.
19. Joseph Pizzorno, "Glutathione!" *Integrative Medicine: A Clinician's Journal* 13, no. 1 (February 2014): 8–12, https://www.ncbi.nlm.nih.gov/pmc/articles/PMC4684116/.
20. Ibid.
21. Deanna M. Minich and Benjamin I. Brown, "A Review of Dietary (Phyto) Nutrients for Glutathione Support," *Nutrients* 11, no. 9 (September 2019): 2073, https://doi.org/10.3390%2Fnu11092073.
22. Ibid.
23. Weidong Qi et al., "Quercetin: Its Antioxidant Mechanism, Antibacterial Properties and Potential Application in Prevention and Control of Toxipathy," *Molecules* 27, no. 19 (October 2022): 6545, https://doi.org/10.3390%2Fmolecules27196545.
24. Ibid.
25. De Oliveira et al., "Effects of Quercetin on Polychlorinated Biphenyls-Induced Liver Injury in Rats."
26. Jiri Mlcek et al., "Quercetin and Its Anti-Allergic Immune Response," *Molecules* 21, no. 5 (May 2016): 623, https://doi.org/10.3390%2Fmolecules21050623.
27. Cleveland Clinic, "What Selenium Is and Why You Need It (But Not Too Much of It)," May 31, 2023, https://health.clevelandclinic.org/selenium-benefits/.
28. P. D. Whanger, "Selenium in the Treatment of Heavy Metal Poisoning and Chemical Carcinogenesis," *Journal of Trace Elements and Electrolytes in Health and Disease* 6, no. 4 (December 1992): 209–21, https://pubmed.ncbi.nlm.nih.gov/1304229/.
29. Masaaki Nakamura et al., "Methylmercury Exposure and Neurological Outcomes in Taiji Residents Accustomed to Consuming Whale Meat," *Environment International* 68 (July 2014): 25–32, https://doi.org/10.1016/j.envint.2014.03.005.
30. A. A. Khalaf et al., "Protective Effects of Selenium and Nano-Selenium on Bisphenol-Induced Reproductive Toxicity in Male Rats," *Human & Experimental Toxicology* 38, no. 4 (December 2018): 398–408, https://doi.org/10.1177/0960327118816134.
31. Xuejiao Zeng et al., "The Protective Effects of Selenium Supplementation on Ambient PM2.5-Induced Cardiovascular Injury in Rats," *Environmental Science and Pollution Research* 25, no. 22 (August 2018): 22,153–62, https://doi.org/10.1007/s11356-018-2292-8.
32. Maryam Sahebari, Zahra Rezaieyazdi, and Mandana Khodashahi, "Selenium and Autoimmune Diseases: A Review Article," *Current Rheumatology Reviews* 15, no. 2 (2019): 123–34, https://doi.org/10.2174/1573397114666181016112342.
33. National Institutes of Health, "Selenium," April 15, 2024, https://ods.od.nih.gov/factsheets/Selenium-HealthProfessional/.
34. Susan J. Hewlings and Douglas S. Kalman, "Curcumin: A Review of Its Effects on Human Health," *Foods* 6, no. 10 (October 2017): 92, https://doi.org/10.3390%2Ffoods6100092.
35. Ibid.
36. Guifang Zhao et al., "Antagonizing Effects of Curcumin against Mercury-Induced Autophagic Death and Trace Elements Disorder by Regulating PI3K/AKT and Nrf2 Pathway in the Spleen," *Ecotoxicology and Environmental Safety* 222 (October 2021): 112529, https://doi.org/10.1016/j.ecoenv.2021.112529.
37. Sheril Daniel et al., "Through Metal Binding, Curcumin Protects against

Lead- and Cadmium-Induced Lipid Peroxidation in Rat Brain Homogenates and against Lead-Induced Tissue Damage in Rat Brain," *Journal of Inorganic Biochemistry* 98, no. 2 (February 2004): 266–75, https://doi.org/10.1016/j.jinorgbio.2003.10.014.

38. J. T. Piper et al., "Mechanisms of Anticarcinogenic Properties of Curcumin: The Effect of Curcumin on Glutathione Linked Detoxification Enzymes in Rat Liver," *International Journal of Biochemistry & Cell Biology* 30, no. 4 (April 1998): 445–56, https://doi.org/10.1016/s1357-2725(98)00015-6.

39. Hewlings and Kalman, "Curcumin: A Review."

40. Maryem Ben Salem et al., "Pharmacological Studies of Artichoke Leaf Extract and Their Health Benefits," *Plant Foods for Human Nutrition* 70, no. 4 (December 2015): 441–53, https://doi.org/10.1007/s11130-015-0503-8.

41. R. Kirchhoff et al., "Increase in Choleresis by Means of Artichoke Extract," *Phytomedicine* 1, no. 2 (September 1994): 107–15, https://doi.org/10.1016/s0944-7113(11)80027-9.

42. Minhee Lee et al., "Artichoke Extract Directly Suppresses Inflammation and Apoptosis in Hepatocytes during the Development of Non-Alcoholic Fatty Liver Disease," *Journal of Medicinal Food* 24, no. 10 (October 2021): 1,058–67, https://doi.org/10.1089/jmf.2021.k.0069.

43. Liangliang Cai et al., "Purification, Preliminary Characterization and Hepatoprotective Effects of Polysaccharides from Dandelion Root," *Molecules* 22, no. 9 (August 2017): 1409, https://doi.org/10.3390/molecules22091409.

44. Cleveland Clinic, "Can You Eat Dandelions?" July 21, 2021, https://health.clevelandclinic.org/dandelion-health-benefits/.

45. Valter D. Longo et al., "Intermittent and Periodic Fasting, Longevity and Disease," *Nature Aging* 1, no. 1 (January 2021): 47–59, https://doi.org/10.1038%2Fs43587-020-00013-3.

46. Davina Derous et al., "The Effects of Graded Levels of Calorie Restriction: XI. Evaluation of the Main Hypotheses Underpinning the Life Extension Effects of CR Using the Hepatic Transcriptome," *Aging* 9, no. 7 (July 2017): 1,770–804, https://doi.org/10.18632%2Faging.101269.

47. Francoise Wilhelmi de Toledo et al., "Safety, Health Improvement and Well-Being During a 4- to 21-Day Fasting Period in an Observational Study Including 1,422 Subjects," *PLoS One* 14, no. 1 (January 2019): e0209353, https://doi.org/10.1371%2Fjournal.pone.0209353.

48. He Wen et al., "Enhanced Phase II Detoxification Contributes to Beneficial Effects of Dietary Restriction as Revealed by Multi-Platform Metabolomics Studies," *Molecular & Cellular Proteomics* 12, no. 3 (March 2013): 575–86, https://doi.org/10.1074%2Fmcp.M112.021352.

49. American College of Healthcare Sciences, "The Hidden Dangers in Your Dietary Supplements," blog, December 2, 2016, https://achs.edu/blog/2016/12/02/dangerous-supplement-ingredients/.

50. Evan L. O'Keefe et al., "Circulating Docosahexaenoic Acid and Risk of All-Cause and Cause-Specific Mortality," *Mayo Clinic Proceedings* 99, no. 4 (April 2024): 534–41, https://doi.org/10.1016/j.mayocp.2023.11.026.

51. Hao Chen et al., "Omega-3 Fatty Acids Attenuate Cardiovascular Effects of Short-Term Exposure to Ambient Air Pollution," *Particle and Fibre Toxicology* 19, no. 1 (February 2022): 12, https://pubmed.ncbi.nlm.nih.gov/35139860/.

52. Noha Gamal Bahey, Hekmat Osman Abd Elaziz, and Kamal Kamal Elsayed Gadalla, "Potential Toxic Effect of Bisphenol A on the Cardiac Muscle of Adult Rat and the Possible Protective Effect of Omega-3: A Histological and

Immunohistochemical Study," *Journal of Microscopy and Ultrastructure* 7, no. 1 (January 2019): 1–8, https://doi.org/10.4103/jmau.jmau_53_18.
53. Institute for Natural Medicine, "Are You Getting Enough Omega-3s?" January 22, 2020, https://naturemed.org/are-you-getting-enough-omega-3s; and Haiyan Tong et al., "Omega-3 Fatty Acid Supplementation Appears to Attenuate Particulate Air Pollution–Induced Cardiac Effects and Lipid Changes in Healthy Middle-Aged Adults," *Environmental Health Perspectives* 120, no. 7 (July 2012): 952–57, https://pubmed.ncbi.nlm.nih.gov/22514211/.
54. Jacob M. Hands et al., "A Multi-Year Rancidity Analysis of 72 Marine and Microalgal Oil Omega-3 Supplements," *Journal of Dietary Supplements* 21, no. 2 (September 2023): 195–206, https://www.tandfonline.com/doi/abs/10.1080/19390211.2023.2252064?journalCode=ijds20.
55. Bonny Burns-Whitmore et al., "Alpha-Linolenic and Linoleic Fatty Acids in the Vegan Diet: Do They Require Dietary Reference Intake/Adequate Intake Special Consideration?" *Nutrients* 11, no. 10 (October 2019): 2365, https://doi.org/10.3390/nu11102365.
56. Angel Gil, Julio Plaza-Diaz, and Maria Dolores Mesa, "Vitamin D: Classic and Novel Actions," *Annals of Nutrition and Metabolism* 72, no. 2 (January 2018): 87–95, https://doi.org/10.1159/000486536.
57. "Time for More Vitamin D," *Harvard Health Publishing*, September 1, 2008, https://www.health.harvard.edu/staying-healthy/time-for-more-vitamin-d.
58. National Institutes of Health, "Vitamin D," September 18, 2023, https://ods.od.nih.gov/factsheets/VitaminD-HealthProfessional/.
59. Angela M. Leung, Lewis E. Braverman, and Elizabeth N. Pearce, "History of U.S. Iodine Fortification and Supplementation," *Nutrients* 4, no. 11 (November 2012): 1,740–46, https://doi.org/10.3390%2Fnu4111740.
60. Chirag M. Vyas et al., "Effect of Multivitamin-Mineral Supplementation versus Placebo on Cognitive Function: Results from the Clinic Subcohort of the COcoa Supplement and Multivitamin Outcomes Study (COSMOS) Randomized Clinical Trial and Meta-Analysis of 3 Cognitive Studies within COSMOS," *American Journal of Clinical Nutrition* 119, no. 3 (March 2024): 692–701, https://doi.org/10.1016/j.ajcnut.2023.12.011.
61. Kenji Oishi et al., "Effect of Probiotics, *Bifidobacterium breve* and *Lactobacillus casei*, on Bisphenol A Exposure in Rats," *Bioscience, Biotechnology, and Biochemistry* 72, no. 6 (June 2008): 1,409–15, https://doi.org/10.1271/bbb.70672.
62. Shivani Popli Goyal and Chakkaravarthi Saravanan, "An Insight into the Critical Role of Gut Microbiota in Triggering the Phthalate-Induced Toxicity and Its Mitigation Using Probiotics," *Science of the Total Environment* 904 (December 2023): 166889, https://doi.org/10.1016/j.scitotenv.2023.166889.

Chapter 9: The Three Ss to Detoxify

1. Kathleen Mikkelsen et al., "Exercise and Mental Health," *Maturitas* 106 (December 2017): 48–56, https://doi.org/10.1016/j.maturitas.2017.09.003.
2. "Exercise & Fitness," *Harvard Health Publishing*, https://www.health.harvard.edu/topics/exercise-and-fitness.
3. Tinsay Ambachew Woreta, "Detoxing Your Liver: Fact versus Fiction," Johns Hopkins Medicine, https://www.hopkinsmedicine.org/health/wellness-and-prevention/detoxing-your-liver-fact-versus-fiction.
4. Joseph Pizzorno, "Glutathione!" *Integrative Medicine: A Clinician's Journal* 13,

no. 1 (February 2014): 8–12, https://www.ncbi.nlm.nih.gov/pmc/articles/PMC4684116/.
5. Benjamin Gollasch et al., "Maximal Exercise and Plasma Cytochrome P450 and Lipoxygenase Mediators: A Lipidomics Study," *Physiological Reports* 7, no. 13 (July 2019): e14165, https://doi.org/10.14814/phy2.14165.
6. Kirstin Lane, Dan Worsley, and Don McKenzie, "Exercise and the Lymphatic System: Implications for Breast-Cancer Survivors," *Sports Medicine* 35, no. 6 (2005): 461–71, https://doi.org/10.2165/00007256-200535060-00001.
7. Shailendra Mehta, "A Study to Assess the Effectiveness of Rebounding Exercise on Lymphedema," *Indian Journal of Physical Therapy and Rehabilitation* 6, no. 1 (June 2017), http://ijptr.net/a-study-to-assess-the-effectiveness-of-rebounding-exercise-on-lymphedema-shailendra-mehta/.
8. Perri Ormont Blumberg, "Bouncing Your Way to Better Health," *New York Times*, November 11, 2022, https://www.nytimes.com/2022/11/11/well/move/trampoline-exercise-health-benefits.html.
9. Knuvul Sheikh, "Can Exercise Strengthen Your Immunity?" *New York Times*, September 7, 2022, https://www.nytimes.com/2022/09/07/well/move/exercise-immunity-covid.html.
10. Michael Gleeson et al., "The Anti-Inflammatory Effects of Exercise: Mechanisms and Implications for the Prevention and Treatment of Disease," *Nature Reviews Immunology* 11 (August 2011): 607–15, https://www.nature.com/articles/nri3041.
11. Stoyan Dimitrov, Elaine Hulteng, and Suzi Hong, "Inflammation and Exercise: Inhibition of Monocytic Intracellular TNF Production by Acute Exercise via β2-adrenergic Activation," *Brain, Behavior, and Immunity* 61 (March 2017): 60–68, https://doi.org/10.1016/j.bbi.2016.12.017.
12. Wiley Barton et al., "The Microbiome of Professional Athletes Differs from That of More Sedentary Subjects in Composition and Particularly at the Functional Metabolic Level," *Gut* 67, no. 4 (March 2017): 625–33, https://gut.bmj.com/content/67/4/625.
13. Barbara Benham, "Weight-Loss Surgery May Release Toxic Compounds from Fat into the Bloodstream," *Hub*, November 15, 2019, https://hub.jhu.edu/2019/11/15/toxins-in-bloodstream-after-bariatric-surgery/.
14. Eleonora Rotondo and Francesco Chiarelli, "Endocrine-Disrupting Chemicals and Insulin Resistance in Children," *Biomedicines* 8, no. 6 (May 2020): 137, https://doi.org/10.3390/biomedicines8060137.
15. Kumail K. Motiani et al., "Exercise Training Modulates Gut Microbiota Profile and Improves Endotoxemia," *Medicine & Science in Sports & Exercise* 52, no. 1 (January 2020): 94–104, https://journals.lww.com/acsm-msse/Fulltext/2020/01000/Exercise_Training_Modulates_Gut_Microbiota_Profile.11.aspx.
16. "Exercising for Better Sleep," Johns Hopkins Medicine, https://www.hopkinsmedicine.org/health/wellness-and-prevention/exercising-for-better-sleep.
17. Ibid.
18. Danielle Pacheco and Abhinav Sing, "Exercise and Sleep," Sleep Foundation, October 11, 2023, https://www.sleepfoundation.org/physical-activity/exercise-and-sleep.
19. Stephen J. Genuis et al., "Human Elimination of Phthalate Compounds: Blood, Urine, and Sweat (BUS) Study," *Scientific World Journal* 2012 (2012): 615068, https://doi.org/10.1100/2012/615068.
20. Aly Cohen and Frederick vom Saal, *Non-Toxic: Guide to Living Healthy in a Chemical World* (Oxford, UK: Oxford University Press, 2020).

21. Wen-Hui Kuan, Yi-Lang Chen, and Chao-Lin Liu, "Excretion of Ni, Pb, Cu, As, and Hg in Sweat under Two Sweating Conditions," *International Journal of Environmental Research and Public Health* 19, no. 7 (April 2022): 4323, https://doi.org/10.3390%2Fijerph19074323.
22. Genuis et al., "Human Excretion of Bisphenol A."
23. Joy Hussain and Marc Cohen, "Clinical Effects of Regular Dry Sauna Bathing: A Systematic Review," *Evidence-Based Complementary Alternative Medicine* (April 2018): 1857413, https://doi.org/10.1155%2F2018%2F1857413.
24. Jari A. Laukkanen and Tanjaniina Laukkanen, "Sauna Bathing and Systemic Inflammation," *European Journal of Epidemiology* 33, no. 3 (March 2018): 351–53, https://doi.org/10.1007/s10654-017-0335-y.
25. Hussain and Cohen, "Clinical Effects of Regular Dry Sauna Bathing."
26. Oliver Cameron Reddy and Ysbrand D. van der Werf, "The Sleeping Brain: Harnessing the Power of the Glymphatic System through Lifestyle Choices," *Brain Sciences* 10, no. 11 (November 2020): 868, https://doi.org/10.3390%2Fbrainsci10110868.
27. Mark Michaud, "Not All Sleep Is Equal When It Comes to Cleaning the Brain," University of Rochester Medical Center, February 27, 2019, https://www.urmc.rochester.edu/news/story/not-all-sleep-is-equal-when-it-comes-to-cleaning-the-brain.
28. Ursula Prosenc Zmrzljak and Damjana Rozman, "Circadian Regulation of the Hepatic Endobiotic and Xenobitoic Detoxification Pathways: The Time Matters," *Chemical Research in Toxicology* 25, no. 4 (April 2012): 811–24, https://doi.org/10.1021/tx200538r.
29. Vincent Soreca, "Sleep-Wake Disturbance Highly Prevalent in Populations with Liver Disease," Gastroenterology Advisor, September 24, 2021, https://www.gastroenterologyadvisor.com/liver/sleep-wake-disturbance-highly-prevalent-in-populations-with-liver-disease/.
30. Suzanne Leigh, "Depression, Anxiety May Take Same Toll on Health as Smoking and Obesity," University of California, San Francisco, December 17, 2018, https://www.ucsf.edu/news/2018/12/412676/depression-anxiety-may-take-same-toll-health-smoking-and-obesity.
31. Annelise Madison and Janice K. Kiecolt-Glaser, "Stress, Depression, Diet, and the Gut Microbiota: Human–Bacteria Interactions at the Core of Psychoneuroimmunology and Nutrition," *Current Opinion in Behavioral Sciences* 28 (August 2019): 105–10, https://doi.org/10.1016%2Fj.cobeha.2019.01.011.
32. Robert H. Shmerling, "Autoimmune Disease and Stress: Is There a Link?" *Harvard Health Publishing*, October 27, 2020, https://www.health.harvard.edu/blog/autoimmune-disease-and-stress-is-there-a-link-2018071114230.
33. Ting-Ting Li et al., "Effect of Breathing Exercises on Oxidative Stress Biomarkers in Humans: A Systematic Review and Meta-Analysis," *Frontiers in Medicine* 10 (April 2023): 1121036, https://doi.org/10.3389/fmed.2023.1121036.
34. J. David Creswell et al., "Brief Mindfulness Meditation Training Alters Psychological and Neuroendocrine Responses to Social Evaluative Stress," *Psychoneuroendocrinology* 44 (June 2014): 1–12, https://doi.org/10.1016/j.psyneuen.2014.02.007.
35. Omar Hahad et al., "Environmental Noise-Induced Effects on Stress Hormones, Oxidative Stress, and Vascular Dysfunction: Key Factors in the Relationship between Cerebrocardiovascular and Psychological Disorders," *Oxidative Medicine and Cellular Longevity* 2019 (November 2019): 4623109, https://doi.org/10.1155/2019/4623109.

36. Cohen and vom Saal, *Non-Toxic*.
37. Stephanie Dutchen, "Noise and Health," *Harvard Medicine*, Spring 2022, https://magazine.hms.harvard.edu/articles/noise-and-health.
38. Ibid.
39. Hahad et al., "Environmental Noise-Induced Effects."
40. Dutchen, "Noise and Health."
41. Joel M. Lerner, "A Good Wall, Even If It's Made of Plants, Can Reduce Highway Noise," *Washington Post*, March 11, 2005, https://www.washingtonpost.com/archive/realestate/2005/03/12/a-good-wall-even-if-its-made-of-plants-can-reduce-highway-noise/07eaa1fe-3397-4d26-a959-1f3d15029b7a/.

The *Detoxify* Plan

1. Stephen A. Goutman et al., "Residential Exposure Associations with ALS Risk, Survival, and Phenotype: A Michigan-Based Case-Control Study," *Amyotrophic Lateral Sclerosis and Frontotemporal Degeneration* 25, nos. 5–6 (April 2024): 1–11, https://doi.org/10.1080/21678421.2024.2336110.
2. Richard Pullicino et al., "A Review of the Current Evidence on Gadolinium Deposition in the Brain," *Clinical Neuroradiology* 28, no. 2 (June 2018): 159–69, https://pubmed.ncbi.nlm.nih.gov/29523896/; and Francesca Arena et al., "Gadolinium Presence, MRI Hyperintensities, and Glucose Uptake in the Hypoperfused Rat Brain after Repeated Administrations of Gadodiamide," *Neuroradiology* 61, no. 2 (February 2019): 163–73, https://pubmed.ncbi.nlm.nih.gov/30377745/.
3. Emmeline Lagrange and Jean-Paul Vernoux, "Warning on False or True Morels and Button Mushrooms with Potential Toxicity Linked to Hydrazinic Toxins: An Update," *Toxins* 12, no. 8 (July 2020): 482, https://doi.org/10.3390/toxins12080482.

About the Author

Dr. Aly Cohen is a triple board-certified physician in rheumatology, internal medicine, and integrative medicine and one of the country's leading medical and legal experts in environmental health. She gives lectures around the country on environmental health for universities, medical schools, and physician-training programs, and is on the faculty of the Academy of Integrative Health & Medicine, Southern California University of Health Sciences, and the University of California, Irvine, where she creates and manages environmental medicine and integrative rheumatology curriculum for doctors and researchers. She is the coauthor of the bestselling consumer guidebook *Non-Toxic: Guide to Living Healthy in a Chemical World* and co-editor of the textbook *Integrative Environmental Medicine*, part of the Oxford University Press/Weil Integrative Medicine Academic Series. In 2015, she launched The Smart Human, a social-media-based health education platform and podcast designed to empower people to make safer, smarter lifestyle choices to reduce their chemical exposure and increase their overall well-being. Dr. Cohen also appears frequently as an environmental health expert for national news outlets and has given TEDx talks, published peer-reviewed medical articles, acted as a legal medical expert on exposure cases, and collaborated with the Environmental Working Group, Cancer Schmancer, Environmental Health Trust, and other top disease-prevention organizations. With degrees from the University of Pennsylvania and the Hahnemann University School of Medicine (now Drexel University), Dr. Cohen has also received a number of awards for her work in health education, including the Burton L. Eichler Award for humanitarianism. Today, Dr. Cohen continues to see patients in her medical practice in Princeton, New Jersey, where she lives on a farm with her husband, two sons, and lots of furry friends.

You can follow Dr. Cohen's environmental health information and tips on her social media platform, The Smart Human.

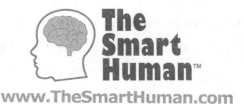

www.TheSmartHuman.com

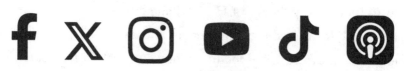